# TAI
# CHI

QIGONG

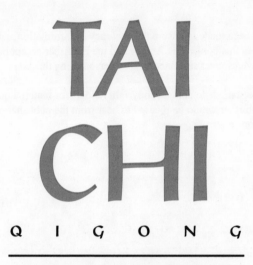

# TAI CHI

## QIGONG

### For Stress Control and Relaxation

## Senior Master Gary Khor E.A.

FOUNDER AND PRESIDENT
OF THE AUSTRALIAN ACADEMY OF TAI CHI

HEIAN

Every attempt has been made to ensure the accuracy of information and the safety of instructions given in this book. The Author and the Publisher accept no responsibility for any injury whatsoever sustained by any person using this book.

Every effort has been made to contact copyright holders for material quoted. The Author and the Publisher would be pleased to hear from the publisher or author to rectify any omissions or errors.

TAI CHI FOR STRESS CONTROL AND RELAXATION

© Gary Khor, 1993

First published in Australia in 1993 by
Simon and Schuster Australia

First American Edition 1994 by
**Heian International, Inc.**
**1815 W. 205th St. Ste.# 301**
**Torrance, CA 90501**

Khor, Gary, 1947-
   Tai chi for stress control and relaxation
   Bibliography.
   Includes index.
   ISBN 0-89346-795-2
   1. Tai chi chuan.  2.  Stress management.  3.  Relaxation - Technique.
   1. Title.

Illustrations by Leslye Cole
Designed by Michelle Havenstein

Printed in Singapore

# Foreword

Stress, it's often thought, is part of modern urban living. But it's hard to imagine a more stressful life than living in the time of the cave-person. The struggle for food, shelter and comfort, which, for the most part is expected as a given in modern Western societies, was complicated by the need for protection; protection against pestilence, plague, famine and war. The human (and indeed animal) response to these stressors was twofold; 'flight', or the physical removal of oneself from the situation, or 'fight', or the physical removal (or attempt thereof) of the stressor.

As the saying goes, 'the more things change, the more they stay the same'. Stress is still a problem. It's the way an individual responds to a situation, rather than the situation, per se. And as long as there are people, there will therefore always be stress. The ways of coping with this — 'flight' and 'fight' — are also still the same (with the possible addition, according to Dr George Sheehan, of 'negotiation'). Only the stressors have changed. As a result, coping has become harder. If it's the boss or the spouse who's causing angst, it's not so easy to run away, or get physical. The only answer is to 'escape'; either by physically removing oneself from the stressful situation, or doing so mentally.

Tai Chi is one of those masterful Eastern techniques with centuries of development behind it. It combines both the physical and mental means of 'escape' that help to restore order and 'control' to a hectic life. As such it represents one of the most effective ways of not only dealing with stress, but building a positive foundation for health-related behaviour.

Gary Khor has been one of the leaders of Tai Chi instruction in Australia. We first met on a Chinese cruise ship when I was in charge of fitness — conditioning bodies for their life back home — and he was in charge of Tai Chi — conditioning minds. Our meeting changed my outlook (and I think his) and exposed for us both the old philosophical conundrum that mind and body are best when joined rather than disconnected. Tai Chi does that and Gary Khor's book on the subject explains this in easily understandable terms.

*Garry Egger MPH, PhD*

*Centre for Health Promotion and Research,*
*Sydney and Discipline of Behavioural*
*Sciences in Medicine, Faculty of Medicine,*
*University of Newcastle*

# Contents

# Introduction

Tai Chi's relaxation, health maintenance and healing benefits have been known and enjoyed by the Chinese for more than 700 years. Recently, Tai Chi's 'secrets' have begun to filter into the West, bringing a new approach to health, well-being and even happiness.

*Tai Chi for Stress Control and Relaxation* unlocks, what are for us, the mysteries of this ancient art. In contrast to traditional Western medicine, Tai Chi recognises the interdependence of mind, body and spirit. Its gentle exercises bring balance and harmony, and allow the *chi* to flow.

The Chinese understand *chi* as 'life-force', and regard the free-flowing movement of *chi* throughout the body as essential for a healthy life. Stress is the major factor which can block the flow of *chi*, but the slow and gentle movements of Tai Chi can remove stress and replace it with relaxation. Only when you are relaxed can you function at your optimum level.

I have written *Tai Chi for Stress Control and Relaxation* so that you too can experience and enjoy the benefits of Tai Chi. Based on my 20 years of experience teaching Tai Chi in Australia, I have modified traditional Tai Chi exercises so that they slowly introduce Tai Chi to people unfamiliar with it. As Tai Chi is also for the mind, I have also explained the history, philosophy, principles and techniques behind the art.

Chapter One examines our own Western lifestyle — often fast-paced, demanding and highly stressful — and explores the mental and physical effects such a lifestyle can have on you. It then shows you how the dynamic meditation, movement and breathing of Tai Chi work to overcome stress.

Chapter Two gives you a better understanding of how and why Tai Chi developed, and how the principles and techniques of Tai Chi promote well-being.

With clear and detailed instructions and diagrams, Chapter Three shows you how to perform the Tai Chi movements.

Chapter Four explains how Tai Chi affects specific parts and functions of your body, and how the movements work to benefit you.

Finally, Chapter Five reveals how the philosophy, principles and benefits of Tai Chi can influence your life. The balance and harmony Tai Chi brings to your mental and physical state can permeate all aspects of your life.

With a relaxed body and a calm and open mind you will be better able to cope with, and perhaps even overcome, the stresses you face. Tai Chi can help you gain balance, health, happiness and peace of mind. All you need do is begin. I hope this book will inspire you.

Gary Khor

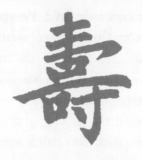

# CHAPTER ONE

# Why Tai Chi?

There can be few people in Australia today who do not spend a good deal of their time feeling tense, rushed and exhausted. Particularly for city-dwellers, the hectic pace of modern living and lack of exercise leave us tired and drained. Most evenings all we want to do is flop down on the sofa in front of the television, blotting out responsibilities, worries and stresses with escapist entertainment and pampering ourselves with sweet treats and snacks.

Rare is the person who, at the end of the day, feels peaceful and content, who actually wants to use their mind, their imagination or their creativity to enrich their lives with a good book, a creative hobby or pursue a whole new area of interest. We have neither the physical energy nor the mental space to live (as opposed to exist) beyond the relentless demands of work, housework, shopping, taking care of children and so on. No wonder that so many of us do so little to improve the quality of our lives! Apart from the requirements of everyday living, there is a tremendous demand on us in terms of time and increased efforts to keep up with changes, deal with constant pressure, and cope with fear of failure.

You may think that none of the above applies to you, that it is an exaggerated scenario. You think you have your life under pretty good control: you know where you are going and what you are doing, that you are doing more than simply coping. Indeed, that's how many of us feel — until we suddenly find we have high blood pressure, or we start suffering migraine headaches or inexplicable digestive problems, or, more commonly, we find we cannot face a single new burden (such as taking on a new area of responsibility at work or organising a big family celebration or caring for a sick relative). Suddenly we feel out of control and at the whim of some giant force that is pushing us around, with no regard for our needs and wishes. In other words, we feel over-stressed.

In order to discover just how stressed you are, compare how you feel day-to-day with how you feel when you go on holiday. At the beginning of the holiday you experience the euphoria of not having to go to work, of travelling to another town or another country, of being with old friends and meeting new people. Instead of being in an air-conditioned office, receiving tense business phone-calls and dealing with unpleasant work problems, or worrying about whether the children have clean clothes for school or whether the car needs servicing, you begin to experience and enjoy the simple things of life: being in the fresh air, feeling the sunlight and the breeze on your face, having the time and the mental energy to talk and have fun with the people you love, being nice to complete strangers, rediscovering the character traits and interests that make you special, individual, unique.

In other words, you reach a state in which stress no longer holds you in a vice-like grip, and you gradually come to the conclusion that you are living your everyday, non-holiday life in a way that you really do not like. You begin to consider ways of getting a job in that foreign city, establishing a business in that small coastal town, buying a small self-sufficiency farm in that glorious rainforest area, in the belief that changing your circumstances in this way will enable you to remain a whole, functioning human being.

Then you go back to work. Sure, the calmness and 'centredness' you found on your holiday remain with you for a while: you are able to deal easily with the irritations and problems of everyday life without feeling overwhelmed and dominated by them. However, this mental and emotional strength rarely lasts for more than six weeks and, inevitably, your life returns to hectic normality. You look back with a certain wistfulness on the time when you felt in control of your life and could enjoy all the small moments of your day. The dream of 'escaping' or of changing your life so that you are in control, inexorably fades.

If this course of events is not what happens to you when you go on holiday, then you must be dealing exceedingly well with the stress in your life. But for most of us it is all too familiar!

Of course, you probably already know the theory of how you could cope better with everyday life: become physically fitter and thus reduce any stress you may feel. This involves attending to your physical, mental, emotional and spiritual needs. Yet it is hard to know exactly what to do, let alone to actually do it.

We all know, for example, that we should exercise at least three times a week, and some of us (albeit a small minority) do actually play sport or get other exercise on a regular basis. Most of us exercise only erratically. For a few months or years we become addicted to, say, jogging, aerobics or muscle-building, but then give up on it when faced by setbacks or difficulties, however much good we feel the exercise may be doing us. Or, simply, we get bored by the exercise: our bodies may be exercising, but our minds remain unsatisfied. Or we train too hard, sustaining injuries that preclude doing that sport for a while, thus eroding our determination and sapping our will. Once that happens, exercise becomes too much like hard work, so we give up.

Given that most of us cannot substantially change our lives (by, for example, being able to give up work) and so remove many of the stresses we face, what we need to do is change the way we live day to day.

You need some form of exercise that gently and steadily exercises and relaxes the body and, most importantly, refreshes the mind. You need to be able to control the stress you are experiencing, instead of being controlled by it. You need to develop your spiritual and emotional resilience so that you can put the demands and stresses of life in proper perspective and not be overwhelmed by them. You need to prevent health problems before they happen. As a highly beneficial daily health-care program best known for its relaxing effects, Tai Chi can help you achieve well-being and balance in your life.

A recreational exercise art which has been practised by the Chinese people for more than 700 years, Tai Chi is a system of flowing movements for exercising and developing the body and mind. Its basis lies in a philosophy derived from the principles of nature, which place it in harmony with the needs of our minds and bodies, rather than at odds with them, as are so many other forms of exercise.

Before we explore in detail how Tai Chi works and how to perform it, we need to look carefully at what causes so many of our physical, emotional, psychological and spiritual problems: STRESS. Without understanding what the problem is, we cannot fully understand how to fix it.

## THE STRESS OF LIFE

Everybody has it; everybody talks about it; yet few have taken the time to find out what stress really is.

We often look back longingly to a time when we imagine that the human race had no stress, but in fact human beings have always been subject to stress of one kind or another. Yet with each generation, complexity and additional stress are added to our lives. The technological advances of the last hundred years, particularly the last fifty, are supposed to have made life easier, but paradoxically they have intensified the stress in our daily existence, mainly by increasing expectations and standards of performance. No longer is it enough, for example, to keep the house clean, the clothes washed and food on the table: we feel compelled to keep the house looking like a magazine advertisement, the clothes whiter than white and completely wrinkle-free and to cook food of gourmet standard. Washing machines and microwave ovens, computers and facsimile machines may have taken the drudgery out of work but they have also moved expectations and goals even further out of reach.

Stress is a part of our lives which, though it can be overcome, cannot be avoided. Indeed, it is very often a topic of conversation: the stress of living in a recession, executive life, unemployment, retirement, exercise, family problems, pollution, the death of relatives or friends. Even schoolchildren are placed under enormous stress, caused by a host of factors such as parental expectations, fear of unemployment in the future, and peer pressure, to name but a few.

## WHAT IS STRESS?

It is hard to define exactly what stress is as the word 'stress', like 'success', 'failure' or 'happiness', means different things to different people. Is 'stress' really a synonym for 'distress'? Or is it effort, fatigue, pain, fear, the need for concentration, the humiliation of censure or even an unexpected great success which requires complete reformulation of one's entire life? The answer to all the questions is yes and no. That is what makes the definition so difficult. Every one of these conditions (and a thousand more) produces stress, but none can be singled out as being *it*, since the word applies equally to all the others.

The word itself comes from the Latin *strictus*, meaning 'to draw tight'. The word 'stress' then became absorbed into the old French word *estrecier*, meaning 'to straighten or narrow'.

These meanings accurately describe what actually happens to your body when you experience excess stress. Your muscles and fasciae (connective tissue) tighten, you tend to hold your limbs and torso straighter and your blood vessels narrow. These are the characteristics of your natural 'fight or flight' response, the condition that enabled primitive humans either to stand and confront danger or to flee it.

During your lifetime you will face a range of totally different problems, but medical research has shown that in many respects the body responds in the stereotyped manner outlined above, undergoing identical biochemical changes which are essentially designed to cope with any type of increased demand upon the human machinery. In other words, although stress-producing factors (technically called stressors) are different, they all elicit essentially the same biological stress response (illustrated in Figure 1, see page 12).

Short-term arousal due to stress can be life-saving, but long-term arousal can be damaging to health as the body's strength is continually drained at a higher rate than normal and no time to recoup energy is given. Long-term depression and feelings of being unable to cope, which may result from prolonged stress, produce slightly different changes and it is thought that they may have even greater potential to be damaging.

The distinction between stressor and stress was perhaps the first important step in the scientific analysis of this most common biological phenomenon that we all know only too well from personal experience. Dr Hans Selye, an internationally acknowledged authority on understanding stress, defines stress as a 'non-specific response of the body to any demand made on it'.

In his book, *Stress without Distress*, he explains that each demand made upon your body is, in a sense, unique — that is, specific. When cold, you shiver to produce more heat and the blood vessels in your skin contract to hold in the heat. When hot, you sweat because the evaporation of perspiration has a cooling effect. When you eat too much sugar and your blood-sugar level rises above normal, you excrete some of it and burn up the rest so that the blood sugar returns to normal. Similarly, any drugs or hormones you take have their own specific effects (and side-effects) on your system.

No matter what kind of derangement is produced, all these stressors have one thing in common: they increase the demand for readjustment. Therefore, although the cause and consequent reaction may be specific, the demand itself is *non-specific*, requiring adaptation to a problem, irrespective of what that problem may be. This non-specific demand for activity is the essence of stress.

Studies show that many maladies have no specific single cause but are the result of a constellation of factors (such as inherited or environmental factors) among which non-specific stress often plays a decisive role. We have to consider that such ailments as peptic ulcers, high blood pressure, nervous breakdown, and so on, may not be primarily due to such causes as diet, genetics, or occupational hazards. They may simply be the products of the ongoing non-specific stress that results from attempting to endure more than we can.

It now seems that 'working hard' or 'getting the job done' are not the prime cause of heart attacks. The culprit is, in fact, the negative thoughts we carry: anger, frustration, tiredness, depression and so on.

Thus, instead of undergoing complicated drug therapies or surgical operations, we can often help ourselves better by establishing whether or not the decisive cause of our illness is stress, which may stem from our relationship with a member of our family or our employer, or it may merely be due to our own over-emphasis on being right every time.

Anything which upsets the balance of the mind or body can cause stress. For the purpose of definition, let us say that 'stress' is 'imbalance' as the stress-response forces the body's functioning into an excited, imbalanced state.

## CAUSES OF STRESS

We all react differently to different potential stressors. One person's mild stimulation from life is another person's intolerable burden. What is severely stressful for one person may be no more than a tiresome niggling incident to another. The degree of stress you experience is determined not simply by external events but by how you perceive the event and respond to it.

The way in which you perceive and respond to a potential stressor is called 'stress motivation'. There are four identifiable categories of stress motivation: cognitive, emotional, psycho-dynamic and situational.

### Cognitive Stress

A natural phenomenon of the human brain is the constant chattering (talking to ourselves) that goes on inside our head.

However, few people are aware that what we say to ourselves has a strong bearing on our mental well being.

If you tell yourself that a particular situation is hopeless, or that there is no way out, it will more than likely end up that way. Also, worrying that something will not work out as you would like causes anxiety and even harmful distress.

Less destructive, but still unsatisfactory, is a much used half-hearted attempt: 'I will try to do my best'. The correct self-talk is 'I will do the best I can'. A positive, self-assertive statement is more likely to get the job done, and thereby help you to avoid a lot of unnecessary stress.


## Emotional Stress

Frustration is another common phenomenon we face in our daily lives. The resultant emotional stress can lead to maladaptive behaviours which make us even more ineffective to handle the cause of the frustration.

When faced with a frustrating and stressful situation we may repeat negative behaviours because they are familiar. Another response includes anger and irritation — not a relaxing response and one which probably will not calm an already tense situation. Both these responses simply compound the initial stress.


## Psycho-dynamic Conflicts

When you are under stress you are quite likely to do over and over again the things that got you into trouble in the first place.

This unconscious preoccupation with past events can keep you in the same stressful situation, and even aggravate it further and thus intensify your stress.

When your proper perception of a situation is blocked by stress, you may not see that you need to respond to the problem differently than you have in the past. Instead, you replay past responses, becoming frustrated and further stressed when these methods don't prove effective. (Also, it is easier to use an old method of coping rather than to try a new one, particularly when you are under stress.)

## Situational Stress

This is imposed upon us by the physical environment and takes many forms: crowding, sudden or repetitive noise, cold, heat, and so on.

## Life's Stressful Events

Various events in everyone's lives commonly cause stress. The following list includes some of the most stressful events.

- Death of a spouse or partner
- Divorce
- Separation from spouse or partner
- Death of a close family member
- Gaol term
- Personal injury or illness
- Marriage
- Fired from employment
- Marital reconciliation
- Retirement

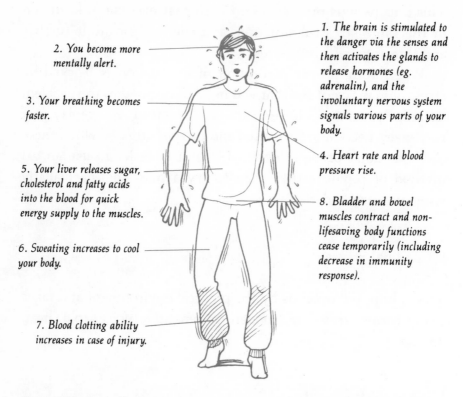

2. You become more mentally alert.

3. Your breathing becomes faster.

5. Your liver releases sugar, cholesterol and fatty acids into the blood for quick energy supply to the muscles.

6. Sweating increases to cool your body.

7. Blood clotting ability increases in case of injury.

1. The brain is stimulated to the danger via the senses and then activates the glands to release hormones (eg. adrenalin), and the involuntary nervous system signals various parts of your body.

4. Heart rate and blood pressure rise.

8. Bladder and bowel muscles contract and non-lifesaving body functions cease temporarily (including decrease in immunity response).

**Figure 1 The Stress Response**
The 'Fight or Flight' response produces a chemical cocktail to activate your system when you are faced with a stressful situation. Short term, this response can be lifesaving. Long term, it can be damaging to your health.

## THE STRESS RESPONSE

From our primitive ancestors we have inherited a remarkable capacity to arouse and energise the brain and the body in the service of superb performance. We can prime and focus our physical and mental resources to respond quickly to a challenge or threat.

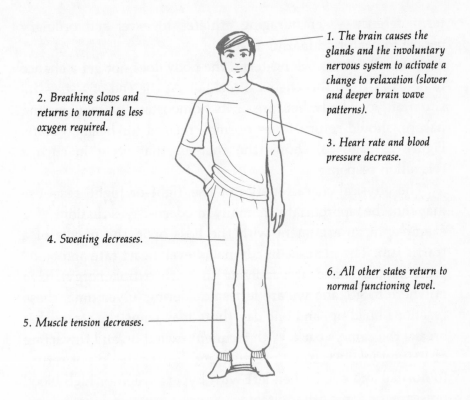

1. The brain causes the glands and the involuntary nervous system to activate a change to relaxation (slower and deeper brain wave patterns).

2. Breathing slows and returns to normal as less oxygen required.

3. Heart rate and blood pressure decrease.

4. Sweating decreases.

6. All other states return to normal functioning level.

5. Muscle tension decreases.

*Figure 2 The Relaxation Response*
*The relaxation response is what happens when the stressor is removed or the attention of the mind is shifted to a relaxing or pleasing thought or image. It is the detoxifying response your body must achieve after a stressful situation if it is to remain healthy.*

The 'fight or flight' response produces a chemical cocktail to activate your system when you are under stress. The adrenal glands produce the hormone adrenalin to stimulate your system, and the pituitary, thyroid and pancreas glands also secrete their own hormones. The effects of these chemicals being released are shown in Figure 1. These chemical reactions can be a source of great strength given the right situation — that is, short-term defence — encouraging athletes to excel and ordinary people to perform amazing feats.

Yet if the stress is long-term, the body does not get a chance to detoxify from this chemical cocktail. At the end of a stressful situation your body, because of its homeostatic or rejuvenating nature, should return to its normal, relaxed (or healing) state. Figure 2 (page 13) shows the changes that occur in such a relaxation response.

The physical characteristics of the 'fight or flight' response may not be appropriate in many modern-day situations, for example, in an argument with the boss or in the middle of a traffic jam. The increase in adrenalin level, heart rate and blood pressure (all aimed at supplying us with extra energy) have nowhere to go, and we are left smouldering. Over time, these reactions build up, and one day there may come the straw that breaks the camel's back. With frequent excitation and thwarting of natural instinct, blood pressure and heart rate do not return to normal and one is then left with hypertension or high blood pressure, or some other disease.

Also, the production of the cortisone hormone becomes a threat. (Cortisone lessens the immune system's response so that the body can receive more energy.) Indeed, medical experts estimate that 50–70 per cent of all diseases are at least partially caused by stress. It would therefore seem a matter of survival that you learn how to control and manage your stress.

## RECOGNISING THE WARNING SIGNS OF STRESS

Each person tends to have his or her own pattern of stress response, so that warning signs of stress vary from person to person. There are many signs that a person is under stress.

One of the most obvious and early signs of stress to look out for is an intensification of personality traits. The suspicious person becomes defensive; the careful becomes over-meticulous; the pessimistic, lugubrious; the anxious, panic-stricken; the inadequate falls to pieces altogether. The irritable person becomes explosive; the extrovert becomes slapdash; and the introspective loses contact with everyday reality.

However, perhaps the earliest and most apparent warning sign is an exaggeration of eating habits. Some people lose their appetite when they become stressed, anxious or depressed; others eat more or over-eat, perhaps to comfort themselves.

To know the pattern of your own stress response is a step forward, for you can then gauge the depth of problems by the nature and severity of your own symptoms or changes in behaviour.

Stress warning signals include:

- Feeling unable to slow down or relax
- Explosive anger in response to minor irritation
- Anxiety or tension lasting more than a few days
- Inability to focus your attention
- Fatigue
- Sleep disturbances
- Tension headaches
- Cold hands or feet
- Aching neck and shoulder muscles
- Indigestion
- Loss or increase of appetite
- Diarrhoea or constipation
- Ulcers
- Heart palpitations
- Allergy or asthma attacks

Although we all experience some of these symptoms at various times for various reasons other than stress, be alert if the symptoms occur frequently. However, it is important not to panic, as this in itself will cause stress.

## STRESS-MOTIVATED BEHAVIOUR

We all wish to learn how to deal with stress. We don't like the experience and want to get rid of it — just as when we itch, we scratch; when we have a headache, we take an aspirin; when we have indigestion, we take antacids. Anyone who has suffered migraine headaches, chronic allergies or nagging arthritis can attest to the extreme measures we use to achieve relief.

How we attempt to achieve relief from mental or emotional stress can take many forms. For the purpose of illustration, here are two classic examples.

Consider the story of a domineering woman who couldn't abide her husband's habit of cracking his knuckles. It caused her so much stress that she moved out of home and eventually divorced him. However, she felt lonely living alone and so married another man — who then developed a habit of grinding his teeth.

Now consider the case of a father whose son died of leukaemia. After nearly two years, the father's grief was still unremitting. He couldn't change the situation, so he focused on the stress itself: he tackled the problem of the stress and not the grief that was the cause of it. This man learned to confine his grief to times of quiet and private contemplation.

He still grieved, but the stress no longer absorbed his energy or constricted his view of the world.

These two examples illustrate behaviours which were induced by stress — the first behavioural response was not effective in dealing with the stress, the second was. Had the wife in the first story recognised her own responsibility for her stress, life may have been less disruptive. Instead of aggravating her stress with anger, a more constructive approach would have involved calming herself and letting go of the stress.

When you feel stressed, it is important that you correctly determine what the cause is. Often it is our own reaction, rather than the situation itself, which aggravates instead of relieves any tension we may be feeling. When a stressful situation cannot be changed easily, the stress itself must become the focus of change. This is what Tai Chi can help you achieve.

## IS STRESS A SIGN OF WEAKNESS?

Many people fear that stress is a sign of weakness, an umbrella for hysterics and malingerers, an excuse that trendies and yuppies give for not being able to cope with 'the real world'. Some hide or deny their stress and its symptoms, afraid of being labelled a bludger or a wimp. Yet wherever people live and work, there will be stress; and no-one is immune to it.

Employers are often reluctant to talk about stress, worried that even mentioning the subject will create a 'bandwagon' effect, with everyone using it as their excuse not to perform. Parents avoid discussing it, for fear of putting dangerous thoughts into adolescent minds.

The result of such avoidance, however, is that stress and its effects are usually dealt with after the event, when the damage has already been done. Yet with intolerable stress, *a pinch of prevention is worth a kilo of cure.*

## IS STRESS ALWAYS HARMFUL?

Where there is no stress there is no life and, certainly, not all stress is bad. A minimum level of stress or stimuli is necessary for life and growth. Too little stress in your life has several adverse effects.

With no stress at all the systems of your mind and body tend to deteriorate and stagnate. Just as excess stress from over-exercise weakens your body's ability to withstand infection, so your capacity to resist disease falls if there is not a minimum level of exercise. Worse, your body loses the capacity to respond to even normal stresses. Lie in bed for several weeks and even the simple act of walking can seriously stress your system.

At the other end of the stress continuum, stress can be tied up as much with challenge and excitement as with anxiety and depression, but it comes in many guises. For example, when deadlines are pressing and solutions cannot be found, stress creates no pleasure; and the stress of such excessive or chronic anxiety is always harmful.

However, when opportunities are evident and rewards are imminent, the stress of an identical situation can create joy. The positive stress of challenge and excitement fuel the forces of achievement. The stress of appropriate, well-balanced exertion gives rise to health, fitness and well-being.

Stress is a powerful servant but a tyrannical master. It can be a rich source of energy in the service of achievement and creativity, or it can be a source of corrosion and exhaustion. It can be a cause of illness, or a force for health. Your reaction to it is what gives it positive or negative power over your life.

## TAI CHI AND STRESS MANAGEMENT

As we have seen, there are many ways to become stressed, but when most of us talk about stress today we usually talk about being mentally stressed, and these mental worries, fears and frustrations of each day spilling over into our physical system. While non-mental forms of stress can be simply attended to by removing the stressor, such as the heat or cold or noise, mental stress is another matter. Yet, just as in a condition of excess heat we create behaviours and systems that can reduce the heat, so too can we create techniques and behaviours that reduce the mental stress that is affecting us.

Tai Chi enables you to do just this. The technique it uses to dissipate mental stress consists of two processes: first it relaxes the mind and allows the flowing movements to reduce the stress put into the physical system and, second, it removes the physical effects of the stress itself.

Rocks are hard and unyeilding
The rivers flow around them and forget.

Tai Chi's flowing movements and 'energy meditations' have the therapeutic effect of slowing down the pace and refreshing the body with peaceful relaxation and renewed energy. Tai Chi relaxes the mind and body, quiets the nervous system, benefits the heart and blood circulation, cures indigestion, loosens stiff joints, tones up muscles and refreshes the skin. It re-establishes balance, both physically and mentally, encouraging your body and mind to return to their rested states.


## HOW TAI CHI WORKS

The three main aspects of Tai Chi are meditation, movement and breathing. These subjects are fully detailed in subsequent chapters, but a basic understanding of their role in Tai Chi is essential before you read any further.


### Tai Chi and Meditation

The word 'meditation' confuses or scares many Westerners because it implies 'meditating' on some profound but perpetually obscure idea that is never quite defined to anyone's satisfaction. In fact, meditation is one of the most ancient and most common of human activities.

Whether you realise it or not, you are probably already very familiar with the 'meditative mood'. Just think of times when you feel relaxed; when your mind drifts far away, contemplating pleasant images or thoughts, and when a good feeling rests within you. You could be lying on the grass, looking at the sky, making pictures in the clouds and then watching them drift by. You could be sitting on the beach, watching the movement of the ocean, and listening to the sound of the waves as they flow in and out. When you feel the sun shining on you, its warmth mirroring the warm, comfortable feeling inside you . . . All these simple examples reveal the meditative mood.

Experiencing such moments of inner stillness is vital to your mental and therefore your physical well-being. In its normal state the mind is a constant source of mental activity, a never-ending network of thought associations. Just stop for a moment and try to think of nothing. Impossible, isn't it?

In the endless sea of thoughts, the mind gets no rest. Even in sleep, unfinished business from the day is played out in dream fantasies. In stressful situations, such as the break-up of relationships or financial difficulties, the turmoil is increased. We have natural safety valves such as sleep, leisure, sports, hobbies and, to a certain extent, daily chores, but these are not enough, so residual pressure continues to build up inside. Meditation has proved to be one of the most effective ways of relieving this pressure.

In essence, meditation consists of concentration and relaxation: your mind focuses on an object while your body relaxes in a comfortable position. This is made easiest by having a passive attitude and a quiet environment. The basic aim is to silence the thinking mind (the inner chatter) and shift the awareness from the rational to the intuitive mode of consciousness.

In many forms of meditation this silencing of the rational mind is achieved by concentrating one's attention on a single item, like one's breathing, the sound of a mantra (a repeated word or phrase), or the visual image of a mandala (a circle which is a symbolic depiction of the psyche or self). Yet these can be difficult techniques to learn.

Tai Chi, however, is one of the most pleasurable forms of meditation. Its flowing movements and mental visualisations of each exercise give it an extra dimension which is not present in the static forms of meditation. (Visualisation is further discussed in Chapter 2, pages 45 to 47.)

## Tai Chi and Movement

Once you calm and focus your mind, you can begin to relax. When you control your thoughts as well as your actions, making them one of the same thought or image, you bring your mind and body into balance and harmony. There is no longer any conflict and you can relax.

Balance and harmony are reflected in Tai Chi movements. There is the shifting of the body weight from one foot to the other and the series of continuous, light, subtle transitions between forward and backward movements, emptiness and fullness and so on. Each limb movement is accompanied by movements of the whole body, and muscles and bones are brought into an orderly action of withdrawals and extensions. The continuous, soft and circular movements of Tai Chi bring about continuity and then calmness and relaxation.

The slowness of Tai Chi teaches balance through muscle control and coordination. It also allows you more time to be aware of each action and, with conscious control of the movement, prevents damage to muscle tissue from sudden exertion. Visually, Tai Chi resembles an effortless dance, but in reality every movement is performed with a great deal of internal strength and control.

Tai Chi movements tone, stretch and exercise every muscle of your body. You will gain physical, mental and spiritual benefits, and an overall feeling of vitality.

## Tai Chi and Breathing

When performing Tai Chi, correct breathing is vital to gaining maximum benefit from the movements. Your aim is to gain control of your body's functioning to allow it to receive the physical benefits of the rested state. The physical activity of proper breathing has psychological as well as physiological benefits — it reduces your metabolic rate, thus making you feel more relaxed.

Correct breathing is abdominal breathing. To breathe abdominally, you need to use your diaphragm, not just your chest, which allows only shallow breathing. This breathing technique is detailed fully in the following chapter, but fortunately there are no complicated techniques to learn as Tai Chi naturally enhances or induces it.

The physical benefits of abdominal breathing are many. By tensing and relaxing your abdominal muscles, the pressure is alternately high and then low. This not only makes the blood within your abdominal cavity flow more smoothly but it also improves the blood circulation of all other organs, especially the liver and spleen, the blood reservoirs of the body. Other organs located near your diaphragm and also affected by its rise and fall include the heart, the lungs, the kidneys, the stomach, the small and large intestine, the gall bladder, bladder and so on.

The movement of your limbs and body in Tai Chi enhances the massaging effect abdominal breathing has on these, some of the most important organs for life.

Breathing is one of the first things affected by stress. In the 'fight or flight' response, your breathing rate speeds up, and the nostrils and air passages in your lungs open wider in order to take in more air as quickly as possible. With sustained stress, your breathing becomes shallow and insufficient oxygen circulates through the body, limiting your energy.

Proper breathing, however, can not only undo many of the stress-related problems you may experience but can also act to reduce the level of mental stress as well. Breathing abdominally during your Tai Chi exercises will help to overcome any stress you may be feeling and thus restore calmness, energy and strength.

## OTHER BENEFITS OF TAI CHI

Certainly, Tai Chi is best known as a way to achieve relaxation and tranquillity: the swimming and weaving motions soothe tired and over-stimulated nerves and relax tense muscles. However, the practical applications of Tai Chi are immense. Some of the better-known applications follow.

As a physical health system, Tai Chi will in time revolutionise the concept of body-fitness exercise. The generally accepted theory of fitness exercise, especially in the Western world, is that we should perform hard and vigorous physical exertion. This often results in painful injuries, permanent damage and uneven body development.

Tai Chi, on the other hand, utilises the principles of non-exertion and internal energy exercises. It teaches the art of flowing movements and gentle relaxing exercises to gradually develop and strengthen the whole body evenly. This rejuvenates the body, and increases your resistance to disease and illness. It also keeps you physically fit, fluid and sensitive.

As a healing art, Tai Chi is widely used by the Chinese to alleviate or, in some cases, cure insomnia, arthritis, rheumatism, anaemia, chronic indigestion, listlessness, mental strain, depression and nervous breakdown.

On an artistic level, Tai Chi movements can be used to enhance a dancer, actor, or masseur's flow and movements, whilst musicians use it for creativity and inspiration.

In the area of personal growth and development the benefits of Tai Chi are fourfold: physical, mental, emotional and spiritual.

Physically, Tai Chi exercises develop your body to its natural potential of health and fitness, coordination in movement, sensitivity and balance. Body control and self-discipline on the physical plane is the first step to growth and development.

Mentally, this 'moving meditation' art, through physical control and stability, creates a balanced mind capable of making rational decisions and taking responsibility. The mind is active, free and spontaneous. Tai Chi energy meditations stimulate and clear the mind. The flowing movements calm the spirit and sharpen the mental faculties, and the mind-directed exercise increases sensitivity and awareness.

Emotionally, Tai Chi is a stabilising force because of the good breathing, proper balance and positive mental state it demands and creates. The physical and mental exercise gives proper channelling to your emotional energy. Further, Tai Chi stimulates and releases 'blocked' energy and facilitates positive expression. (Blocked energy results when muscles are tense and do not allow blood and energy to flow freely through them.)

Spiritually, the philosophy of *yin-yang* balance which is central to Tai Chi is at the core of all growth and development. (The philosophy of Tai Chi is detailed in the following chapter.) The balance of *yin* and *yang*, of positive and negative, calms and stabilises the mind. This calmness will enable you to examine your life from a more positive and realistic viewpoint, and give you the will and the way to improve things. (The spiritual benefits of Tai Chi are explored in detail in Chapter 5.)

## WHO CAN BENEFIT FROM TAI CHI?

The answer to this question is everyone. Male or female, young or old, unfit or superfit, people with or without disabilities, Tai Chi has something to offer you.

Unlike some forms of exercise, Tai Chi does not adversely affect a woman's hormonal cycle and, in fact, can improve it. If you are getting on in years then Tai Chi allows you to enter exercise at your own health level without risk. The same goes for those who are unfit and for anyone with a physical or mental disability.

Even if you are superfit Tai Chi can improve your coordination and help to remove stress. It can teach you to use your body efficiently and avoid damaging techniques. It is also a perfect system for warming up before sport.

*IMPORTANT POINTS*

- Stress is a natural part of our everyday life.

- Stress can affect our physical health, and long-term stress can be damaging.

- Stress is an imbalance, caused by anything that upsets the balance of the mind or body.

- The degree of stress is determined by how a person perceives an event and responds to it.

- When a stressful situation cannot easily be changed, the stress itself must become the focus of change.

- With intolerable stress, a pinch of prevention is worth a kilo of cure.

- We must exercise gently and steadily, relaxing the body and refreshing the mind.

- Tai Chi movements reduce physical stress, remove its effects and stimulate and clear the mind.

- Tai Chi gradually develops and strengthens the whole body evenly.

- The benefits of Tai Chi are physical, mental, emotional and spiritual.

- Everyone can benefit from Tai Chi.

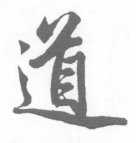

CHAPTER TWO

# *The Philosophy and Principles of Tai Chi*

## ORIGINS OF TAI CHI

In order to be able to perform Tai Chi effectively, it is necessary to understand something of its origins and the philosophy from which it developed. Without such knowledge, you would benefit from only the physical aspect of the exercises (and then only minimally), for it is your coordination of body and mind that is the key to performing and benefiting from Tai Chi.

Woven into the fabric of this subtle art — its graceful and relaxing exercises making it appear deceptively simple — are the timeless wisdom and health secrets of the Chinese people: their philosophies, customs and traditions; their beliefs; their healing systems; and, finally, the Chinese mind, which has shaped and moulded Tai Chi into what it is today.

The art and philosophy of Tai Chi are derived and synthesised from three main sources: the collective philosophies of the ancient Chinese, Shaolin martial art and the study of nature.

## ANCIENT PHILOSOPHIES

The aims of the ancient philosophies that have influenced and shaped Tai Chi are manifold, ranging from the purely physical to the social, the spiritual and, some would say, the supernatural. Let us consider briefly the major influences.

### Lao Tzu and Taoism

Lao Tzu (born 604 BC) taught the doctrine of the Tao (pronounced 'dow') or Naturalism, which is drawn mainly from the recognition of the soft, yielding ways of nature. Amongst other things, he formulated three major principles that are central to Tai Chi.

First, according to Tao, it is only by observing, learning from and conducting our lives according to the ways of nature that we can expect to reach a state of fulfilment and peace. You should do nothing that conflicts with the natural way: you should bend with the wind and become a part of it, rather than attempt to resist. A snow-covered leaf does not resist, but bends slowly and gracefully until the snow falls away. It does not obstruct, fight or confront the snow but, instead, submits to its greater force and ultimately triumphs.

According to the laws of nature, nothing is permanent,

everything is forever changing. Everything is born, it evolves and dies and is reborn again, thus creating a never-ending circle. In effect, there is no beginning and no end. This concept is reflected in the changing seasons.

Also, everything in nature has a complementary or opposite component which is represented by the attributes *yin* and *yang*. For example, hot and cold, night and day, male and female and so on. Through all the changes occurring in nature, harmony is established through the balance of *yin* and *yang*. When *yin* and *yang* are not balanced, disorder occurs. The concepts of *yin* and *yang* are further discussed on pages 33 to 36.

Taoism is in fact the major influencing philosophy of Tai Chi. Taoism regards the physical and spiritual as indivisible yet distinctly different aspects of the same reality, with the body serving as the root for the blossom of the mind. The purpose of Tai Chi is to regain the balance between body and mind to achieve harmony.

The second major principle is the Taoist doctrine of the 'Uncarved Block' which describes humans in a pristine state of existence, before they are tainted by family, education, environment and society, before they are changed by bigotry and greed. To attain fulfilment, each of us must again become pure, virgin, untouched — as an uncarved block. In your heart and mind you should contemplate only those things that accord with the natural laws. Only by doing this can you find peace within yourself.

Third is the doctrine of *Wu Wei*, or 'Non-action', which does not advocate that you should be completely passive, doing nothing or always turning the other cheek, but, rather, that you should do only the things that need to be done and act only in ways that accord with the natural law. It means doing things for their own sake rather than for ulterior motives. Perhaps most importantly, it means knowing when to stop rather than over-doing things. As Lao Tsu made the point:

*When your work is done, then withdraw!*
*That is the way of Heaven.*

The Taoist principles are intertwined directly in the philosophy of Tai Chi. In particular, the doctrine of naturalism influences the movements of Tai Chi and ensures that each applies the concepts of softness, yielding and non-action. This results in the inner calmness and tranquillity of the performer as he or she moves with, rather than attempts to resist, the laws of nature.

Nature constantly changes, and this is reflected in Tai Chi exercises by the constantly changing movements. The shifting of the weight from one foot to the other and the alternating movements of the limbs help to bring balance and harmony.

## Confucius and Confucianism

Confucious (551–479 BC) formulated a philosophy of humanism which concentrates on the world of the living, rather than on life in the next world or on spiritual needs. His doctrines focus on social conduct and order, and ethics and morality in particular.

Confucius taught that the goal of the individual is to cultivate the qualities of social grace, justice and wisdom (with special respect for family elders). His goal for society was universal order and harmony. He also believed in the necessity of reverence and respect for the human body.

The Confucianist philosophy of order and harmony is reflected in the postures and movements of Tai Chi. Tai Chi exercises involve upward and downward, left and right, and forward and backward motion. When these movements are properly balanced, harmony results. Tai Chi promotes harmony within the self and, as a consequence, the ability to deal calmly and fairly with others.

## Buddha and Buddhism

Unlike naturalistic Taosim or humanistic Confucianism, Buddhism is concerned with the after life and the way to the next world.

Buddha (550–477 BC) expounded a philosophy of non-materialism: that all things are transient, that they lack continuous form and have no ultimate content. He preached a doctrine of love and compassion to overcome hatred and revenge. He taught that to find peace, we must learn to conquer the self and extinguish the ego. In this way, we will extinquish the causes of all our suffering: our attachments and desires.

The essence of Buddha's teaching is evident in the non-ego and non-materialistic attitude of Tai Chi philosophy. These aspects are further emphasised in the Tai Chi practice of 'emptying' all stress and tension from the body and mind, resulting in the 'non-action' way of doing things. Tai Chi teaches you to let go of your worries and concerns as you concentrate on the movements you are performing. In this way, it frees you from the constraints of the self.

The Buddhist teaching of proper posture, proper breathing and focusing the mind are also directly reflected in Tai Chi practice.

As well as individual philosophers and their doctrines, the philosophical foundations of Tai Chi encompass the *I Ching*, and the concepts of *yin* and *yang* and *chi* (energy).

## The *I Ching*

The *I Ching*, or *Book of Changes*, is one of the oldest Chinese books of wisdom, dating back some 3000 years. It consists of a series of sixty-four hexagrams and interpretations of them, having originally evolved from ancient divinations, and was one of the first attempts made by humans to explain and rationalise the mystery of the universe.

Originally a manual of oracles, it developed into a book of wisdom from which both the Confucian and Taoist philosophies drew inspiration. The name (as well as the rationale of the book) refers to the concept of constant change, which is the result of the interaction of two complementary forces: *yin* and *yang*.

## The *Yin* and *Yang* and the Five Elements

The ancient Chinese philosophers believed that in the beginning the universe was void and boundless, and they called this state *Wu Chi*. From *Wu Chi* evolved motion, *yang*, and its opposite aspect, stillness, *yin*. The universe was created through the interplay of *yin* and *yang*, and the state which included both these aspects was called Tai Chi.

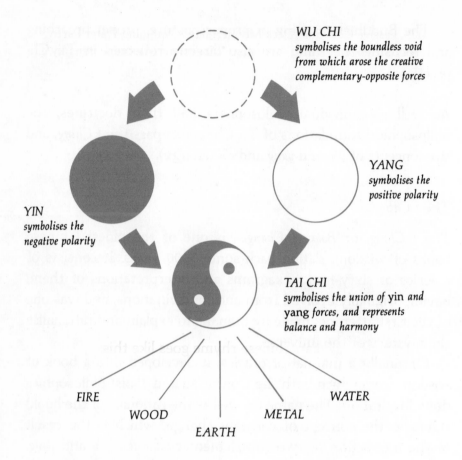

**Figure 3 The Chinese Theory of Creation**
*The Chinese believe that from a state of nothingness (Wu Chi) arose inactivity (yin) and activity (yang). Tai Chi is the union of these two forces, the interaction of which gave rise to the five basic elements: fire, wood, earth, metal and water.*

The concepts of *yin* and *yang,* also provide a means to understand and measure the qualities and characteristics of all things. The opposite and complementary aspects of each are as follows:

34

YIN Passive Cold Soft Dark Moon Stillness Feminine Water Earth
YANG Active Hot Hard Light Sun Movement Masculine Fire Sky

It is important to note that *yin* and *yang* are not labelled good and bad. Instead they have a creative relationship, and are constantly interacting and changing, with one never existing in isolation from the other. This interdependence is illustrated in Figure 3, where a small part of *yin* is found in *yang* and vice versa. As an example: *yin* and *yang* can be related to the negative and positive poles of a current — separate and opposite to each other, yet both part of the whole current. Without them, the current would not exist.

From the interaction of *yin* and *yang* arose the five basic elements: wood, fire, earth, metal and water. These elements can exist in a helpful and complementary relationship to each other, or they can work against one another and destroy themselves. A popular Chinese rhyme goes like this:

> *Wood burns to produce Fire,*
> *resulting in ash which becomes Earth.*
> *From Earth there emerges Metal,*
> *which produces Water by condensation.*

Also:

> *Wood occupies Earth,*
> *and Earth soaks up the Water.*
> *Water douses Fire,*
> *Fire melts Metal,*
> *and Metal cuts Wood.*

The five elements feature in Tai Chi movements, being represented as advance (metal), retreat (wood), shift to the left (water), shift to the right (fire), and central equilibrium (earth).

The concepts of *yin* and *yang* are the foundation of traditional Chinese medicine, which aims to balance the two forces within the body. This engenders equilibrium and harmony as an imbalance in the relative amount of *yin* and *yang* energy causes illness.

The art and philosophy of Tai Chi is based on the interplay and changeability of *yin* and *yang*. This creates a balance of movement and provides grace to the Tai Chi exercises. The harmony which results promotes the holistic benefits of Tai Chi.

## Chi

Another concept crucial to understanding Tai Chi is that of *chi*, or energy, for throughout the practice of Tai Chi runs a central theme: the cultivation, storage and circulation of the *chi* energy in the body. In Chinese this is called *Qigong* (spelt by the ancient Chinese as *Chi Kung*) or energy meditation. Good health depends upon the proper balance and distribution of *chi* throughout the body.

According to the Chinese, the universe, humanity and nature are greatly influenced by *chi*. They believe that the universe and everything in it is derived from *chi*, that it permeates all matter, and regard it as the essential life-force of all living things.

*Chi* literally means air, breath, energy, vapour, gas. Philosophically it can be defined as intrinsic energy, biophysical energy, or the life-force.

The Chinese view *chi* as an invisible energy force which circulates throughout the body to give life. They believe that we are born with a fixed amount of this vital energy, prenatal *chi*, which is stored in the *tan tien* (a psychic energy centre, located three finger widths below the navel). This energy is gradually depleted throughout life, but it is also augmented by energy obtained from food and air, postnatal *chi*.

The energy or *chi* is circulated throughout the body along the various meridians. According to ancient Chinese philosophy, these are the paths along which blood and energy are transported to the organs in an intricate pattern of energy flow circuits.

*Chi* is activated and directed by the mind and is responsible for the movements of the body. In order for *chi* to be effective, it must first be cultivated, and secondly, exercised, so that the body and mind become one with the universe. The various meditation exercises of Tai Chi, aided by the process of respiration, help you to achieve this.

Our personal *chi* is inseparable from the *chi* of the universe, and continually interchanges with it. This reciprocal flowing back and forth is the essence of life. When the flow of *chi* is strong, we are healthy. If the flow is blocked in any area, we become ill. Death occurs when the flow of *chi* stops completely.

The complete renewal of *chi* takes place during deep relaxation (such as during sleep, however, an even deeper state of relaxation is achieved during meditation.) *Chi* of the universe is received by the brain during the period of profound relaxation, when the pattern of the electrical waves continually given off by the brain become regular.

In Tai Chi, the postnatal *chi* is lowered to the *tan tien*, thus lowering one's centre of gravity and establishing a more balanced position. The mind and body become peaceful and tranquil, and all movements become graceful and harmonious. To cultivate consciously the transformation of food and air, by the mind, into *chi*, and to influence consciously the movement of *chi* in the body is the ability Tai Chi will give to you.

Everyone has *chi* power, though it is not developed to the same degree in every individual. Just as we know of the presence of the subconscious mind, so too should we all be aware of the power of *chi*.

## Meridian Theory

As we have seen, fundamental to Chinese philosophy is the concept of energy or *chi*. The Chinese regard every phenomenon of the universe, including humanity, as a manifestation of this energy.

Your own vital energy, *chi*, is conducted through the body in channels or pathways called meridians. These are not blood or nerve systems. Rather they make up an invisible network that links together the fundamental substances (*chi*, blood and fluids) and organs. They connect the interior of the body to the exterior.

The meridian system is made up of twelve regular meridians that correspond to each of the five *yin* and six *yang* organs and to the pericardium (the outer muscle of the heart). There are two other major meridians, the governing vessel, the *du mai*, and the conception vessel, the *ren mai*.

The governing vessel is the central control meridian which governs the *yang* organs. It begins at the *hui yin* point, runs

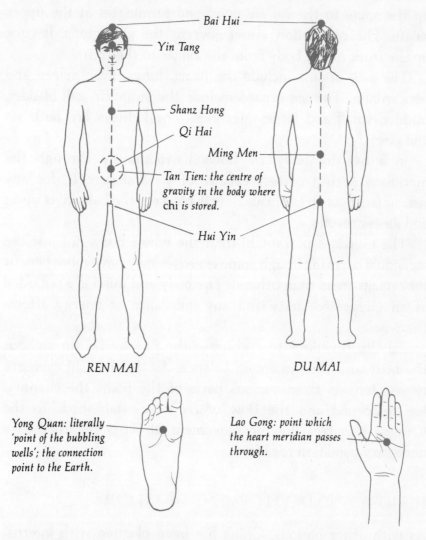

**Figure 4 The Two Major Meridians**

*Your vital energy, chi, is conducted throughout your body via channels or pathways called meridians. These figures illustrate the two major meridians which control all the others. The Du Mai, or governing vessel, controls the* yang *meridians, and the* Ren Mai, *or conception vessel, controls the* yin *meridians.*

up the spine to the *bai hui* point and terminates at the upper palate. The conception vessel governs the *yin* organs. It runs up the front of the body from the *hui yin* to the chin.

The *yang* organs include the heart, lungs, liver, spleen and pericardium. The *yin* organs include the stomach, gall bladder, bladder, small and large intestines. The kidneys are both *yin* and *yang*.

In a healthy body, *chi* flows harmoniously through the meridians with a correct balance of *yin* and *yang*. If, for any reason (such as stress), this flow is blocked, the balance is upset and illness results.

The exercises of Tai Chi treat the whole body, not just the individual parts (although some exercises may have more benefit for certain areas than others). The body and mind are regarded as an integrated unity and any imbalance of energy affects the whole.

Tai Chi functions to encourage the flow of *chi* throughout the body and thus maintain balance. As the Tai Chi exercises release tension from various parts of the body, the channels are re-opened and the flow of *chi* is re-established. To the Chinese this free-flowing movement of *chi* is regarded as a necessary condition for life.

## HISTORY AND DEVELOPMENT OF TAI CHI

As with other nations, China has been plagued with internal wars throughout its history, one dynasty succeeding another. Just as Europe had King Arthur, Charlemagne, Richard the Lionheart, Robin Hood and Joan of Arc, so China has had plenty of heroic emperors, fighting monks and other extraordinary figures in whose exploits fighting skills reached their zenith.

Strongly intertwined with the tradition of fighting is the Chinese preoccupation with the concept of hygiene. Hygiene, as understood by the Chinese mind, is the pursuit of good health and long life. Therefore, both fighting and hygiene work to sustain life, and the quality of life, for those who practise them. This connection provided the foundation for the development of the martial arts, from which Tai Chi evolved.

## The History of Hygiene

The earliest records of the importance and influence of hygiene can be traced to the third millennium BC, when Emperor Fu Hsi introduced his people to a form of medicine for health maintenance. In 2575 BC, the legendary Yellow Emperor, Huang Ti, established a national health program. History records that he also practised a breathing exercise (called *Tu' Na*) and a form of gentle calisthenics (called *Tao Yin*). (He also ritualised a primitive wrestling sport called *Go-ti*).

During the Han Dynasty (202 BC to 220 AD), one of China's greatest physicians, Hua To, introduced the first organised exercise system based on the movements and characteristics of animals. He called his system 'Five Animal Frolics'. The exercises were fashioned on the movements of the bird, monkey, deer, tiger and bear, and so reflect movements found in nature.

## Development of the Martial Arts

The strongest influence on the development of martial arts was a Buddhist monk called Tamo (or Bodhidaruma). In the sixth century AD he arrived at the Shaolin temple in China's Honan province to teach the monks Zen. However, due to their poor physical condition, the monks were unable to stay awake during his classes. So, to improve their health and assist their meditation, he introduced a series of exercises which emphasised rhythmic breathing, coupled with bending and stretching of the body.

Yet, a further benefit to the exercises was to evolve. The presence of marauding outlaws was a constant threat, and the monks were forbidden to use weapons to defend themselves. The necessity of survival caused the Shaolin system to evolve self-defence benefits, and gradually a form of martial art developed. The Shaolin type of combat utilised hard, stiff and sharp punching and kicking movements. It eventually came to be known as the hard or external school of Kung Fu.

In time, the fighting monks of the Shaolin temple gained a feared, yet respected, reputation throughout China. However, as Shaolin Kung Fu reached its zenith, it was to be transcended.

In the thirteenth century, a Taoist monk, Chang San Feng, studied boxing at the Shaolin temple and quickly mastered the skills. However, he observed that the Shaolin style of hard techniques had limitations and that it was not in keeping with the laws of nature.

Chang San Feng's thirst for knowledge and understanding of martial arts pervaded his waking and sleeping hours. A chance observation of an encounter between a snake and a crane inspired his breakthrough and a new approach to the martial art system.

From the twisting, curling, lifting and parrying combatative techniques of the snake and the crane, Chang San Feng realised the value of yielding and changing. These actions corresponded with the principles expounded by Taoist philosophy. The combat of the crane and the snake exemplified to him the principle of the *I Ching*: that is, the strong changing to the yielding and the yielding to the strong. He remembered Lao Tzu's analogy of the yielding water and the hard stone:

> *Nothing under heaven is more*
> *yielding than water; but when it attacks things hard and resistant,*
> *there is not one of them that can prevail!*

Chang San Feng then proceeded to study other animals, trees, water, clouds, and so on, and from these observations he designed an exercise system which includes such movements as 'white crane spreading wings' and 'waving hands in the clouds'. Thus was born the soft or internal school of Kung Fu Tai Chi (properly known as Tai Chi Chuan, which literally means Supreme Ultimate Fist).

Tai Chi, as a form of Kung Fu, incorporates the original definition of *kung fu*: a special skill, an ability, a task or the time involved in any worthwhile art — for example, carpentry, farming, painting, calligraphy and, especially, alchemy. (Eventually the term 'Kung Fu' became a colloquiallism used in reference to any of the Chinese martial arts.)

Tai Chi provides the balance of action and non-action essential for life. This focus developed from China's philosophical history, which revealed the need for *yin* and *yang* balance, as well as from its fighting and health-care history, which showed that in addition to being strong, one also needed to yield to conserve energy — the *chi* or life force.

## THEORY OF TAI CHI

Keeping in mind the philosophies of Tai Chi as you practise will help you to gain maximum benefit from the exercises.

Tai Chi movements are based on the coordination of the mind, the inner body, and the outer body; the intent (*yi*), vital energy (*chi*) and internal strength (*chin*). The mind directs the *chi*, and the *chi* in turn directs the body. The act of performing Tai Chi also involves the circulation of the vital energy (*chi*) and, together with concentration, it produces what the Taoist called Spirit (*shen*).

That Tai Chi is an exercise for both the mind and body can sometimes be overlooked when learning the moves. Therefore in Chapter 3, along with the instructions for each move, I have listed mental imagery which is appropriate to the move.

## PRINCIPLES OF TAI CHI

Now we come to the essential principles in the practice of the art of Tai Chi: relaxation, concentration, meditation, harmony and breathing. You must be aware of these five principles as you practise the movements.

### Relaxation

*Be soft and yielding. Exert no strength.*
Just imagine for a moment that you are about to lift a very heavy box from a table in front of you. Picture the action in your mind but at the same time be aware of how your body feels as you imagine this activity.

Even with no activity occurring at all, you probably tightened your muscles. Perhaps you took in a quick breath of air and then held it, tightening your chest. If you could have measured your blood pressure you would probably have found it rising slightly, with your heart rate increasing. All in all, almost a perfect description of the effects of stress — and achieved simply through imagining a muscular activity!

Now imagine yourself as you are sitting, standing or lying and imagine your body becoming lighter and lighter. First your head seems to lift then your whole body almost drifts away from the ground. Focus on this image for perhaps a minute.

More than likely your muscles became relaxed. Your breathing deepened into continuous steady breaths. Possibly your blood pressure fell marginally. Quite a different scenario from the previous one. Yet, in fact, your body is probably much heavier than the imagined weight of the box. In both examples we imagined moving a heavy object up but in one case we imagined muscle power and became stressed; in the other, we simply relaxed and let something happen.

When you perform your Tai Chi, take this soft approach: allow the move to happen. In Tai Chi you should almost allow yourself to be moved rather than move yourself. The Chinese have many expressions to describe the movement of Tai Chi. To them it is like 'riding the wind' or the 'art of the windblown willow'.

## Concentration

*Let the mind direct the movement.*
As seen in the earlier examples, a task is more easily performed

when you not only relax but also imagine yourself doing it — the key being to *allow* something to happen rather than to *make* it happen. This applies to the movements of Tai Chi, and assists you with performing them easily and with as little effort as possible.

To achieve the mental images of visualisation, you need to concentrate. Concentration should not be thought of as mentally gritting your teeth: this would work against the principle of relaxation. The aim is to quieten the inner chatter of the mind, to free it from its daily worries and concerns, by focusing your thoughts on the Tai Chi move you are performing.

Through visualisation, you will gain a keener awareness of the task at hand and not be distracted by what happened that day at the office or at home. This will enable you to concentrate your energy into what you are actually doing, using only the energy your require and wasting none. Take a camera lens as an example. The lens is no more strained when it is focused than when it is unfocused. It simply gives a clearer picture.

As well as visualisation, concentrating on your breathing and the movement of the *chi* throughout your body helps you to focus your attention on the totality of movement of, and within, your body — you are in control. We have already discussed meridian theory and the paths along which the *chi* flows. Breathing technique is discussed on pages 49 to 55.

Getting that clear picture in Tai Chi initially necessitates breaking the move down into smaller parts (you should practise each stage):

1. Visualise the positions where your feet start and finish.
2. Visualise how your hands move.

3. Then put these two pictures together, discovering how
   your hands and feet coordinate.

Remember, your mental focus should be on picturing the movement, not on getting the movement right. If you focus on trying to get the move right, you set yourself up for the stress of failure. A Tai Chi movement that bears little resemblance to the correct movement but that is performed softly, slowly, smoothly and with good posture can provide considerable health benefits. A Tai Chi move that starts and finishes in the right positions but that is performed stiffly, with force and gritted teeth, is unlikely to provide any benefit and may well contribute to stress.

Most of the Tai Chi exercises, outlined in Chapter 3 of this book, contain visualisations to help you with the shape and form of the movements. The terms used to portray these mental images include 'holding a ball' and 'painting a rainbow'. A couple of the exercises only include a second type of visualisation which indicates where to focus your internal energy. Most exercises indicate both. In both forms the emphasis is on enhancing the beneficial effects of the movement, and the aim is to achieve a balance of mind, body and spirit.

## Meditation

*Balance the movements of the mind, the body and the* chi.

When you are quiet and focused on the movement you are performing, when the soft and slow motion is a reflection of the visualisation in your mind and you feel at ease with the movement, then you have reached the meditative state necessary for the proper performance of Tai Chi.

In this stage, not only have you achieved balance between your mind and body, but you have also tapped into and gained control of your *chi*, your vital energy. In the understanding of the Chinese, body, mind and spirit are one and you are at peace with the universe. This is when the healing qualities of Tai Chi can begin.

In terms of technique, this balance will be reflected in the movements you perform. When we are stressed, we tend to move quickly in uncoordinated jerks. This is because excess tension within the muscles makes coordination very difficult. When we learn to move smoothly and evenly during times of stress we have, in effect, learned how to relax our tense muscles and undo the effects of stress.

To move in this way requires continual awareness (hence the meditative aspects of Tai Chi). The Chinese say that movement should be like the action of reeling silk: if you are not to break the delicate thread, you must be conscious of the manner in which you perform every movement. This alert awareness means that you are not focused on your daily worries and problems, and hence the mental as well as the physical side of stress is relieved.

In your Tai Chi practice, try to eliminate sudden changes in speed and direction. There should be no stopping or starting within the form, only circular changes in direction. To do this, keep the shoulders and elbows down and try to avoid sharp angles in the elbow joint. Do not be afraid to use space in your moves. The closer in that you draw your arms and hands, the more jerky the movement will tend to become.

## Harmony

*When thoughts and movements are in accord, you gain the power to heal.*

Through the unity of mind, body and spirit you acquire in Tai Chi practice, you achieve harmony. This is when you reach an agreement, an accord, or a pleasing arrangement of the various parts of yourself.

Rather than making you oblivious to any tension or pain you may be feeling, your awareness of this unity allows you to identify any remaining areas of tension within your body, for in these places the wave of momentum does not flow.

When we focus on feeling our body as a unity, as a whole, we become aware that each move contains within it a wave of momentum usually starting in the feet, flowing through the body and being released through the hands. To encourage harmony of movement, follow this imagery in your Tai Chi moves:

1. Feel your feet firmly rooted against the earth.
2. Feel the power of the move come from your legs.
3. Feel the power directed by the waist.
4. Express the power in the hands.

Gradually you can begin to remove any blocked tension from your body and in this way bring your whole self into the balanced, harmonised state.

## Breathing

*Breathe naturally through the nose into the abdomen. With the abdomen relaxed tranquillity will prevail.*

Crucial to the proper performance of Tai Chi is correct breathing.

Breathing is essential for life. Just as breath symbolises life or the Spirit in Christian theology, so too does it to the Chinese. As we breathe in air, or spirit, it becomes an intrinsic part of us and we of it — all life is connected by this.

As discussed in Chapter 1 on pages 23 to 24, the benefits of correct breathing are numerous. In your Tai Chi practice, along with helping you to relax, awareness of your breathing helps you to focus the mind and gain control over this essential aspect of life.

Before beginning each session of Tai Chi, take a moment or two to bring your breathing in line with the following principles (you can also use this technique if you are in a stressful situation to remove stress):

1. Breathe deeply but without forcing your breathing.
2. Allow (but do not force) your rate of breathing to slow, reducing the number of breaths taken per minute.
3. Have your mouth gently closed and breathe in and out through your nose.

In fact, you should not commence your Tai Chi set of movements until you are satisfied that your breathing is comfortably relaxed and gentle. Once you start your Tai Chi set forget about your breathing and let your body handle it.

## BREATHING TECHNIQUES

The way in which you breathe is a vital part of your health.

You have already seen how gentle relaxed breathing can help

in stress management, but the question of exactly how you breathe is also very important. So, for example, you should breathe through your nose (rather than through your mouth), in order to reduce your susceptibility to airborne infection; and you should use your entire diaphragm (rather than just your chest) each time you inhale or exhale, in order to maximise the circulation of blood to your internal organs.

In Chapter 4 you will learn the detail of how breathing affects the functioning of your body's defence systems and how it can affect the efficiency of your digestive system. In this section, however, the functioning of the breathing system itself is discussed, for without such knowledge it is difficult to perform the movements of Tai Chi.

## Breathing Through the Nose

Few people are surprised at being told that we should breathe in through the nose, rather than the mouth; most of us are aware that our nose is a filter that reduces the risk of airborne infection. Others may be aware that as the air passes down the nasal passages the body has time to heat the air before it falls on to the sensitive lung tissue. But many of us do not know why we should breathe out through the nose.

The important point here is that the nose acts as a valve: you simply cannot breathe out fast through the nose as you can through the mouth. Since the same volume of air passes through the same limited space on the way in as on the way out, the time taken for inhalation and exhalation tends to be equal, whereas when we breathe in through the nose and out through the mouth the inhalation is much longer than the exhalation. Breathing out through the mouth also tends to be achieved by collapsing the chest rather than lifting the diaphragm. *Breathing through the nose encourages us to take slower, deeper breaths.* Tai Chi encourages balanced harmonious breathing using the diaphragm.

One of the common problems with breathing through the nose is that when you first ask a person to breathe through the nose you are often rewarded with a sound like an old steam train shunting. This sound is an indication that too much force is being used in the breathing. The movement of air through the nose should be soft and quiet.

## Diaphragmatic (Abdominal) Breathing

Once you are able to breathe comfortably through your nose, you should aim to breathe with your whole diaphragm, rather than with just your chest; in other words, with your whole lung area, not just with the top lobes.

### Testing for Diaphragmatic Breathing

First, you must ascertain whether or not you are actually breathing diaphragmatically. This is often not the case, both because of a natural tendency to breathe higher and higher in the chest as we age and because the diaphragm, like any other muscle, is subject to stress which may cause it to be held in a more or less static position. If the diaphragm is working, then it will move downwards as you breathe in. This downward movement causes the abdominal area to be compressed and the abdomen consequently expands (which is why diaphragmatic breathing is also called abdominal breathing). On the out-breath, the diaphragm rises and the abdomen therefore contracts.

Think of a sausage-shaped balloon constricted in the middle so that one side represents the abdominal cavity and the other side represents the thoracic (chest) cavity. If you increase the pressure on one side by squeezing it, the other side expands.

*VIP*

So to test your diaphragmatic breathing, stand quietly with your feet about shoulder-width apart and your knees slightly bent. Place your left hand on the area immediately below the navel and place your right hand on top of your left hand. Check that your back is straight and your shoulders relaxed. Breathe naturally, without forcing, in and out through the nose. If, as you breathe in, you feel your abdomen press against your hand and, as you breathe out, you feel your abdomen contract, then you are breathing diaphragmatically. If not, or if the movment is only slight, then you are breathing higher in the chest and your health will be suffering as a consequence.

Be careful that you do not sway your abdomen forward, to create the illusion of diaphragmatic breathing; it is easy to do this without realising what is happening. To test for this, do the exercise exactly as before, but place the back of the right hand against the small of the back opposite the left hand. As you breathe in you should feel the two hands pushed apart; as you breathe out you should feel the two hands come together.

## Teach Yourself Diaphragmatic Breathing

Assume the previously described posture, then close your eyes and visualise the movement of the air from the tip of your nose along the nasal passages, down the throat and deep into the lungs. Then visualise the flow of the air out of the lungs, up the throat, through the nose to the outside.

It is important that your breathing not be forced: you should be mentally following the air, not herding it along. Visualise the air as a stream flowing into and out of your body. Once you have achieved this visualisation you should mentally project the inward flowing stream to a point at the level of your hands, just below the navel. Remember, do not force it, just visualise.

This imagery will sometimes on its own cause the diaphragm to function. If no change occurs, then as well as continuing the visualisation, physically press your abdomen as you breathe out and release the pressure as you breathe in. You will need to practise this every day, but over a period of a few weeks you should be able to dispense with this physical assistance.

If you are very highly stressed then you may find it quite difficult to get the diaphragm to move, even with the visualisation and exercises. To assist in loosening tension in the diaphragm, gently massage with your fingertips from the sternum (breastbone) out along the underside of the ribs. Use the fingertips in a circling motion moving outward from the sternum, pressing in and under the ribs.

It cannot be emphasised strongly enough that throughout these exercises you should continue to breathe at a comfortable frequency and depth. Do not force and flood the system with oxygen; this is not beneficial and can even be hazardous.

## Exercise to Soften and Slow the Breathing

When you stand quietly just before beginning your Tai Chi movements, close your eyes and visualise a lighted candle the flame of which is about five centimetres (two inches) from the tip of your nose. As you breathe in and out through the nose, do so with such smoothness and gentleness that if the candle were real its flame would not even flicker. Focus especially on the change from inhalation to exhalation and vice versa, as this will make for a gentle, rather than abrupt, change between breathing in and out.

Smooth breathing is another example of the silk-like movement mentioned earlier. Jerky, irregular breathing has all the adverse effects of jerky, irregular movement.

## MOVEMENT REVEALED THROUGH PHILOSOPHY

In his writings contained in the *Tao Te Ching*, Lao Tsu recorded his teachings for posterity.

> *Yield and overcome;*
> *Bend and be straight;*
> *Empty and be full;*
> *Wear out and be new;*
> *Have little and gain;*
> *Have much and be confused.*
>
> *Therefore wise men embrace the one*
> *And set an example to all.*
> *Not putting on a display,*
> *They shine forth.*
> *Not justifying themselves,*
> *They are distinguished.*

> *Not boasting,*
> *They receive recognition.*
> *Not bragging,*
> *They never falter.*
> *They do not quarrel,*
> *So no one quarrels with them.*
> *Therefore the ancients say, 'Yield and overcome.'*
> *Is that an empty saying?*
> *Be really whole,*
> *And all things will come to you.*

The verse quoted here reveals Lao Tsu's philosophy of life: the necessary balance of mind and body (empty and be full); the concepts of *yin* and *yang* which, though different, are inseparable (bend and be straight); and the value of yielding (yield and overcome).

These concepts are revealed in the movements of Tai Chi. As we empty our mind of clutter and our body of tension, we fill ourselves with peace; as we bend and soften our body to follow the natural law, we become strong; and as we yield our mind and body to the *chi*, we allow life-giving energy to flow through us. We become calm and confident that we have the strength to overcome any obstacles we face.

*IMPORTANT POINTS*

- The philosophy of Tai Chi is derived from Taoism, Confucianism, Buddhism, the *I Ching*, the concepts of *yin-yang* and *chi*, Shaolin martial art and the study of nature.

- *Yin* and *yang* are complementary forces which exist in the universe.

- *Chi* is the vital energy or life force within you and all things.

- The meridians are the channels along which *chi* flows.

- Key concepts of Tai Chi are continual change, flowing movements, inner calmness, softness, yielding, proper breathing, *chi*, the interdependence of opposites, and inner strength.

- The five essential qualities of Tai Chi movement are slowness, lightness, clarity, balance and calmness.

- The five essential principles of Tai Chi are relaxation, concentration, meditation, harmony and breathing.

- The mind should be focused on the mental imagery of each move.

- The mind commands, the body obeys.

- Abdominal breathing is essential if you are to obtain the full benefit of your Tai Chi practice.

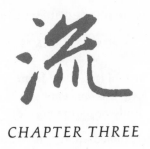

CHAPTER THREE

# Basic Movements

## DEVELOPMENT OF THE BASIC MOVEMENTS

There is an almost infinite number of Tai Chi movements that can be performed, all originally derived from four principal styles that developed over the ages since Chang Sen Feng first drew inspiration from the snake and the crane in the thirteenth century. From these four major styles have come a vast array of different styles, including one very simplified form devised 'for the masses' and promulgated by the Communist government in China. This is the form that is generally performed by large numbers of people morning and evening in town parks and squares throughout China. By and large, however, the Chinese traditionally practise any style of Tai Chi that they choose, modified as necessary to accommodate individual health requirements.

The latest evolution is a style that concentrates on health and philosphy: Tai Chi Qigong Shibashi. The following set of eighteen exercises was developed in China about ten years ago from this form by a traditional Chinese medical practitioner, Dr Chan. His aim was to teach a simple, repetitive (and therefore easy to learn) set of exercises to his patients to use as a means of enhancing their health and longevity. Using knowledge of traditional Chinese medicine and incorporating the continual revelations of Western medical science, I have modified these movements with the aims of:

1. Activating the flow of *chi* along the meridians.
2. Strengthening the internal organs.
3. Increasing longevity by maintaining the health and vigour of the body and mind.
4. Exercising all the joints and muscles.
5. Managing stress by promoting a balanced and relaxed attitude.
6. Preventing occupational diseases such as repetitive strain injury.
7. Promoting postural awareness.
8. Providing the essence and base for many other 'internal' and 'external' martial arts.

This set of exercises is, therefore, a comprehensive health plan designed to cultivate health and energy in every part of the body. It concentrates in turn on all the individual parts of the body, exercising them in carefully graded steps, balancing exertion against relaxation, which is good for reducing stress.

People are used to seeing Tai Chi performed as a continuous flow of movements. Yet, these continuously changing movements prove difficult for beginners to follow. Also, because students are trying to keep up with the form, they often miss out on the essence of the Tai Chi art. One way to avoid this happening is to learn the basics of the art, thereby laying the foundation for the correct practice of Tai Chi.

Simply imitating the form in slow and flowing motion may give you a certain amount of relaxation and exercise for your joints and muscles. However, it does not give you the optimum benefit of your Tai Chi which includes correct posture, abdominal breathing and a focused mind to increase your vitality. These are the three fundamentals of Qigong (spelt as Chi Kung by the ancient Chinese) — the oriental art of energy development.

## BENEFITS OF THE BASIC MOVEMENTS

In essence, these eighteen movements work to increase the body's flexibility, improve abdominal breathing, and focus the mind in meditation. More specifically, if you practise consistently, you will enjoy the following benefits identified by Professor Li Ding, of Shanxi Medical College, China:

Head: your head will feel clear, your body light and comfortable; your memory will increase; you will sleep better, think faster, be more alert and more energetic. These beneficial effects are brought about by the abundance of oxygen supplied to the brain cells and to other cells throughout the body.

Eyes: increased oxygen supply and improved blood circulation help you to see better. When the mind is tranquil, the eyes are bright and the vision clearer.

Heart and lungs: your heart and lung function will improve.

The power of the heart contractions increases; there will be no shortness of breath.

Chest: there will be more cheerful, abundant energy (known as *zhong chi*) in the chest. Your voice will become more forceful and louder, your breathing, smoother and more comfortable.

Spleen and stomach: your appetite will improve, not that you will eat more but that you enjoy what you eat. Nourishment from acquired nutrients will also improve.

Liver and gall bladder: your liver and gall bladder functions will improve, enhancing the digestion and absorption of nutrients, and increasing your body's resistance and immunity to disease. For anyone who often suffers from colds and flu, their occurrence may be prevented or reduced.

Abdomen: fat deposits will be reduced and the peristaltic action of the stomach and intestines improves, making you look better and preventing any increase of cholesterol in the blood.

Reproductive system: increased reproductive ability and also prevention of nocturnal emission, impotence and prostatitis.

Limbs: your joints become smooth and active; the tendons and bones are strengthened; movements become firm and fast.

Spine: its movement becomes smooth and free; hunchback and deformation are prevented.

## HOW TO PERFORM TAI CHI

Immediately before you begin your Tai Chi set, stand quietly for a short time in the preparatory position as outlined on page

65. With your eyes closed, concentrate on your breathing. With your mouth gently closed, breathe deeply but without force through your nose and allow your rate of breathing to slow. Once you are satisfied that your breathing is comfortably relaxed and gentle, put your breathing technique out of your mind and begin the set — your breathing will take care of itself. (Breathing technique is discussed in detail in Chapter 2 on pages 49 to 55.)

When you are learning a movement, practise first the leg-work, then the arm-work, and then put them together with the breathing. Try not to use a mirror to check how you are performing; instead, concentrate on the mental imagery of the movement (and, if you have the opportunity, attend some Tai Chi classes, for these will give you the best indication of how to perform your Tai Chi).

Once you have mastered the individual parts, do each movement once, twice or as often as feels right to you. Then put all the movements together, flowing from one to another in seamless harmony. When you have practised the 'how to' of each movement and can follow the instructions relatively easily, begin your Tai Chi set. Do each movement eight times (four times each side for two-sided movements) or until the movement of the body is rhythmic and coordinated and the mind is in focus. Only by achieving this will you gain the maximum benefit from the movements. For some people this may take fewer than eight repetitions; for others more.

While all Tai Chi moves performed with the Tai Chi principles in mind provide holistic health benefits, the varying nature of each move can be of particular benefit to certain organs, systems and functions. Where there is a specific health benefit in addition to the holistic ones, this has been detailed for you. If you are working on a particular area of your body, you may find it beneficial to visualise that area while performig the move.

It is hard to specify how long the set should take you to perform, for you must develop your own speed or, rather, lack of it. Remember always that the more relaxed you are, the better you will do and the more benefit you will derive. Simply performing slowly is not necessarily the key: deliberate slowness can be just as tension-making as fast movements. Aim always for relaxation.

As a guide, twenty minutes five times a week will maintain and improve your well-being.

---

*IMPORTANT POINTS TO NOTE BEFORE YOU BEGIN YOUR TAI CHI*

- Before starting the set, stand quietly to calm your breathing.

- Breath abdominally, and through the nose.

- Stabilise yourself by lowering your strength from the upper torso into the legs and, even more importantly, lowering the *chi* to the *tan tien* (see Figure 4 on page 39).

- In your posture, elevate the head, hold the neck erect but not tense, and the chin slightly in toward the throat. Let the arms hang freely. Tuck the buttocks in. Do not incline or lean — keep the trunk in a central position.

- In exercises which require turning, turn from the waist, not the knees. Use the waist as the axis of movement. *Turn only as far as is comfortable.* Where degrees of turning are given for specific

---

exercises, these are only meant as a guide — do not strain to these levels. The head should always remain in line with the torso.

- Where you are asked to transfer your weight from one foot to another, move slowly, giving time to make sure the transfer is complete.

- Relax and perform the exercises slowly, smoothly and softly. Balance, coordination and continuous-flowing movements will produce harmony.

- All movements must be controlled by the mind: the mind commands, the body obeys.

- Visualise each movement's imagery as you perform it, and be aware of the movement of *chi* through your body.

- Do each exercise eight times (four times each side in the case of two-sided exercises).

- At the end of the set, stand quietly for a short time in the 'Standing Zen' position.

NOTE these guidelines assume the performer has a healthy body. Where exceptional circumstances arise (such as pregnancy, infirmity, disability, et cetera), please adjust the exercises to suit your needs or, better still, consult your doctor.

## Preparatory Position

The initial or preparatory position for all the following movements is commonly known in Tai Chi as the 'Horse-riding Stance'.

This stance has postural benefits as it encourages an upright spine and relaxes and exercises muscles.

Combined with deep breathing, it also helps to balance the energy of the mind and body.

To achieve the preparatory position:

1. Spread your feet apart, to about the width of your shoulders.
2. Align your toes and heels so that your feet are parallel.
3. Breathe out as you sink down by

**Preparatory Position**
*Place your feet shoulder width apart, and bend your knees slightly to sink down. Your knees should not extend beyond your toes, and your weight should be equally proportioned on each foot. Breathe out while you perform this movement.*

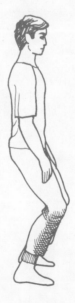

bending your knees slightly. Your knees should not extend beyond your toes.

4. Balance your weight evenly between your feet, making sure that the weight is also equally proportioned on the heel and the ball of the foot.

5. Hold the back straight, keep the head lifted through the *bai hui* point and the tailbone aligned so that the lumbar curvature of the back is not exaggerated.

*MOVEMENT ONE*

# Raising the Arms

This movement is particularly useful in harmonising the cerebral functions of *yi nian* (*yi* refers to willpower, *nian* to intellectual functions such as reasoning and memory).

The movement relieves both physical and mental stress and is good for the joints because it releases their muscular tension and improves circulation of blood and energy to them. There is a good cardiovascular benefit as well and the movement should help normalise blood pressure.

## MOVEMENT BREAKDOWN

### Foot- and leg-work

From the preparatory position, straighten the knees slowly to raise the body, then bend them to sink down.

### Arm-work

Raise both hands to shoulder height in front of you, shoulder-width apart, palms facing down. As you perform the movement, visualise your arms floating, as if they are being drawn up by two floating balloons tied to your wrists.

Next, slowly relax your elbows, then gently press the palms down until your hands are by your sides again. Remember to keep your spine straight.

## Breathing and coordination

Breathe in as you draw your hands up to shoulder height and rise up.

Breathe out as you bend the knees and press down.

## Energy

Focus your mind on the *tan tien* point. As you raise your hands, feel the energy move up the *ren mai* meridian to *shanz hong*. As you let your hands sink, move the energy out along the arms to *lao gong*. In the eight repetitions of the movement keep the focus at *lao gong*.

*1a*

*Breathe in as you rise up and lift your hands to shoulder height in front of you.*

*1b*

*Breathe out as you sink down, relax your elbows and slowly return your hands to your sides.*

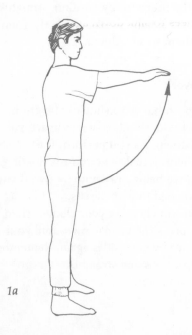

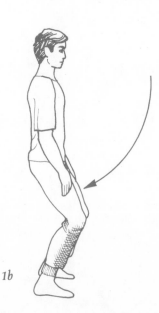

*1a*

*1b*

*MOVEMENT TWO*

# Opening the Chest

The physical expansiveness of this movement has a similar effect on the cerebral functions as 'Raising the Arms'. It is useful in cases of neurasthenia (nervous exhaustion), depression, fearfulness, poor memory, loss of concentration and insomnia.

The increase of oxygen supply to the cerebrum results in clearer thinking and an increase in awareness. This engenders feelings of joy, confidence and general alertness.

## MOVEMENT BREAKDOWN

### Foot- and leg-work

Commence in the preparatory position. Slowly straighten the knees. Then bend the knees to sink down again.

### Arm-work

Raise your hands to shoulder height in front of you, then gently turn them so that the palms face the chest as though you are holding a large ball against you. Keep the shoulders and elbows relaxed.

Now draw the arms out to the sides as far as is comfortable, with palms facing forward.

Bring your hands back into the position of holding the ball, then gently turn them so that the palms face downward, and lower the arms.

## Breathing and coordination

From the preparatory position, breathe in as you straighten the knees, raise your hands and draw them out to the side. The inhalation should be deep, long and slow and the chest should expand as much as possible without there being any forcing.

As you bend the knees, release your breath and return the hands to the holding-the-ball position. Continue to breathe out as you lower the hands.

As you perform the movement, visualise firstly that your arms are embracing a big balloon which, as you breathe in, inflates and pushes your arms to open wider and wider. Then when the balloon reaches its

### 2a
*Breathe in as you rise up and lift your hands to shoulder height in front of you.*

### 2b
*Continue breathing in as you turn the palms to face the chest and then draw your hands out to the side. Remember to keep your shoulders and elbows relaxed.*

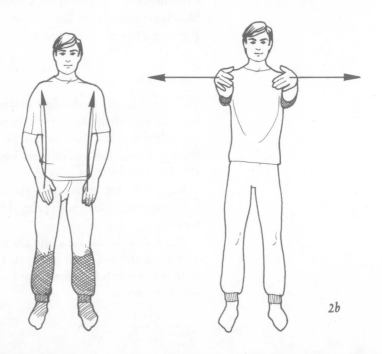

2a

2b

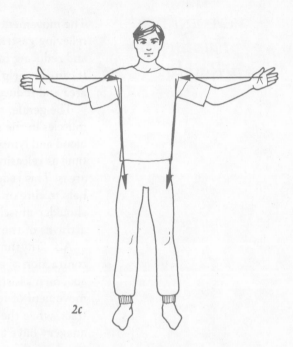

2c

*2c*
*Breathe out as you return your*
*hands to shoulder height in front*
*of you, turn the palms down and*
*lower the arms and sink.*

full size and you let your breath out,
imagine that you are slowly and gently
squeezing it with your arms and body to
push the air out of the balloon.

### Energy

As is Movement 1, the mind should remain
focused on the *lao gong* point.

## MOVEMENT THREE
## *Painting a Rainbow*

The movement is good for digestion, relieving gastric ulcers and stomach-ache, and reducing fat deposits around the waist. It can also help to loosen up the shoulder area and reduce shoulder pain.

The gentle, rhythmic stretching of the muscles in the shoulders and back improves blood and lymph circulation at the same time as releasing tension held in these areas. This reduces muscle fatigue and may help to cure or alleviate lumbar and shoulder-muscle sprains, backaches and arthritis of the shoulder.

Also, rhythmic expansion and contraction of alternate sides of the abdomen assists peristalsis and the movement of food through the alimentary tract, while the deep breathing and relaxed imagery have a positive effect on blood supply to the internal organs.

### MOVEMENT BREAKDOWN

#### Foot- and leg-work

Stand in the preparatory position and shift your body-weight slowly from one leg to the other. Transfer the weight first to the right side, then to the left. When the weight is on the right leg, the right knee should be bent and when the weight is on the left leg, the left knee should be bent.

#### Arm-work

Raise your hands in front of your body and then take them up over the head. Then simultaneously:

1. curve the right hand over the head so that the right palm faces the top of the head. The right elbow is in a gentle curve, the shoulders are relaxed; and

2. lower the left hand down to shoulder height on the left side of the body, palm facing up; at the same time, turn the body to the left so that you can look towards the left palm.

Then simultaneously:

1. Raise the left hand up in a curve over the head so that the left palm faces the top of the head. The left elbow is in a gentle curve, the shoulders are relaxed; and

2. Lower the right hand down to shoulder height on the right side of the body, palm facing up; turn the body to the right and look at the right palm.

As you perform the movement, visualise that your arms are gigantic paintbrushes which you are using to splash colour onto a rainbow, with your fingers as the individual hairs of the brush.

**Breathing and coordination**

Breathe in as you raise the hands over the head.

Breathe out as you shift the weight to the right side, turn to the left and bring the right palm to face the top of the head

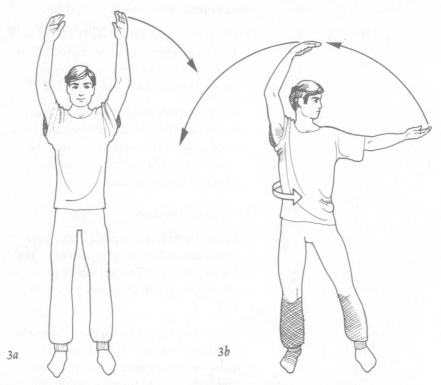

3a

3b

## 3a

*Breathe in as you rise up and lift your hands in front of you until they are above your head.*

## 3b

*Breathe out as you shift your weight to the right, bring your right palm to face the top of your head, turn to the left and lower the left hand.*

*Remember to breathe each time you raise the lowered hand over the head.*

and lower the left hand to shoulder height.

Breathe in as you shift the weight to the left side, turn to the right, raise the left hand over the head.

Breathe out as you lower the right hand.

## Energy

Each time you bring either hand over the head, imagine that the *lao gong* point is filling the *bai hui* point with energy.

## MOVEMENT FOUR
# Separating the Clouds

This exercise improves breathing by exercising the thoracic (chest) muscles. The rising and falling movement of the body stimulates the kidneys, and the motion of the arms improves mobility in the shoulder joints.

The exercise's expansive nature creates a positive mental outlook and improves mental functions generally.

## MOVEMENT BREAKDOWN

### Foot- and leg-work

Stand in the preparatory position and centre the weight between your two feet. Straighten the knees slowly, then bend them slowly. Keep the heels down throughout the exercise.

### Arm-work

Scoop both hands in front of your body, crossing at the wrist so that both palms are facing inwards.

Take the hands up over the head, then turn the palms out and separate the hands, pushing outward imagining that you are separating clouds in the sky.

Then, bring your hands down on both sides of the body until they cross again in front of the abdomen.

Make the separating movement as expansive as possible without straining.

**4a**

*Breathe in as you scoop your hands in front of your body, crossing them at the wrists (palms facing inwards), and then rise up as you take your hands above your head (palms facing outward).*

**4b**

*Breathe out as you sink down and bring your hands down on both sides of your body.*

## Breathing and coordination

Breathe in as you move up, straightening the knees.

Breathe out as you bend the knees and separate and bring the hands down to the side.

## Energy

The focus is again on the *lao gong* point.

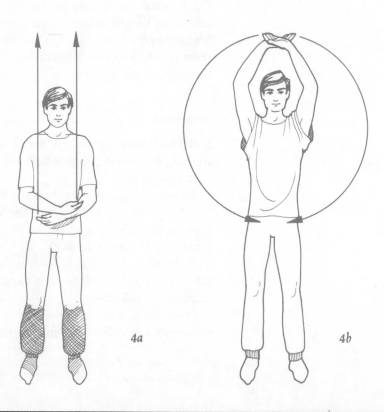

4a                                    4b

## MOVEMENT FIVE
## Rolling the Arms in a Horse-riding Stance

This exercise involves considerable movement of the upper arms and thorax, which improves breathing ability and is recommended to help prevent colds, bronchitis, asthma and the like.

The waist and abdominal movement helps the digestive and excretory functions as well as loosens up the spine.

The joint movements benefit the knees, spine, shoulders, elbow joints and neck.

## MOVEMENT BREAKDOWN

### Foot- and leg-work

Standing in the preparatory position, turn the body to the left. With your knees still bent, turn your body to the right. Turning the waist initiates the movement of the arms.

During these movements, the weight remains centred and does not shift from foot to foot.

### Arm-work

With the arms extended, raise the hands in front of the shoulders. Turn both palms up and draw the left hand down and back, then around in a circle towards the ear and over the shoulder.

Then simultaneously push the left palm forward, and draw the right hand back toward the waist. As the left hand reaches the end of its forward movement, turn the palm to face up. Keep the elbows relaxed and below shoulder level.

TAI CHI FOR STRESS CONTROL AND RELAXATION

Then complete the circular movement of the arm on the opposite side.

The movement of the arms is similar to swimming, except that it is not as large and the palms turn over.

## Breathing and coordination

Breathe in as you bring each hand back. Breathe out as you push forward.

Coordinate the turning of your body with the movement of your hands, for example, when the left hand moves back you should turn slightly to the left.

## Energy

The focus of this movement is at the *lao gong* point, particularly at the moment when the hands pass each other. There should also be a feeling of drawing in the *chi* through one palm and expelling it through the other. There should also be a feeling of drawing energy in through the *lao gong* point as your hand moves backwards, and then releasing energy as you push forward.

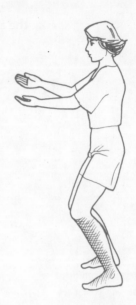

**5a**

*Breathe in as you raise your hands in front of you. Breathe out as you turn the palms up and sink down.*

5a

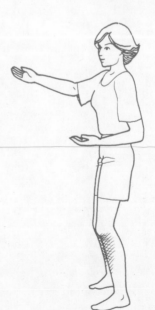

**5b**

*Breathe in as you turn your body slightly to the left and draw your left hand back towards your hip.*

5b

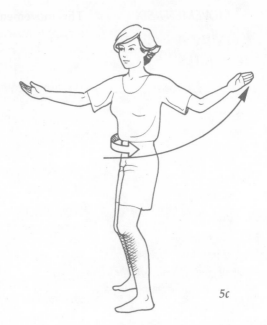

5c

*5c*
*Continue to breathe in as you*
*complete the circular movement*
*of your hand behind your back.*

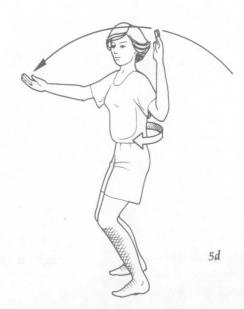

5d

*5d*
*Breathe out as you return to face*
*the front and push forward with*
*your left hand.*

*MOVEMENT SIX*
## Rowing a Boat in the Middle of a Lake

This movement both strengthens the long, straight muscles of the abdomen and internally massages the digestive system and internal organs, improving the functions of the spleen, pancreas and stomach. For this reason it is particularly recommended for those who suffer from indigestion and chronic gastritis.

On a musculo-skeletal basis, it is particularly useful for the hips and shoulders.

**MOVEMENT BREAKDOWN**

**Foot- and leg-work**

From the preparatory position, straighten your knees to rise up, then bend your knees to sink down.

**Arm-work**

Keeping the arms extended throughout the movement, press your hands back behind your body.

In a circular movement, and as though your arms are the oars of a rowing boat, raise your arms upwards and outwards until they are slightly forward of the sides of your body and well above shoulder level.

Press your hands downward as you return them to your sides, completing the movement.

Keep your head erect and your spine straight as you perform the exercise.

*6a*

*Breathe in as you rise up, press your hands slightly behind you and raise them up.*

*6b*

*Breathe out as you sink and, with your arms slightly forward of your shoulders, lower them to your sides.*

## Breathing and coordination

Breathe in as you straighten your knees, take your arms behind you and then raise them up to the front.

Breathe out as you lower the knees and bring the hands down to the sides.

## Energy

The internal focus is at the *lao gong* point.

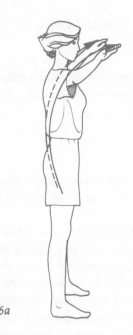

6a

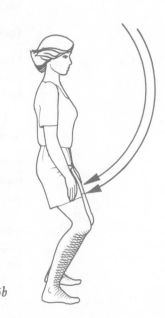

6b

## Supporting a Ball in Front of the Shoulders

This movement improves concentration while reducing stress and tension, especially in the shoulder and lumbar areas. It teaches hand-eye coordination, and is also good for alleviating insomnia and other poor sleeping conditions.

### MOVEMENT BREAKDOWN

**Foot- and leg-work**

From the preparatory position, shift the weight to the right foot and raise the heel of the left foot, simultaneously turning the waist 45 degrees to the right.

Lower the heel of the left foot, then transfer your body-weight to both feet as you return to face the front.

Next, lift the right heel and turn your body 45 degrees to the left.

Transfer your body-weight to both feet as you return to face the front.

**Arm-work**

Lift the left arm upwards across the body so that it finishes palm up in front of the right shoulder, fingers pointing outward. Turn the left palm to face down and then lower the left arm slowly but naturally to the left side.

Then lift the right arm upwards across the body so that it finishes palm up in front of the left shoulder, fingers pointing outward. Turn the right palm to face down and then lower the right arm slowly but naturally to the right side.

As you perform the exercise, visualise when lifting that you are supporting a ball on your upturned palm, and when lowering that you are pressing a ball into water.

### Breathing and coordination

Inhale as you lift the left palm up, lift the left heel and turn the body to the right. Exhale as you turn the palm down, bring the arm to the side, lower the heel and return to face the front.

Then, breathe in as you repeat the movement with your right hand.

### Energy

The internal focus should be at the *lao gong* point.

**7a**

*Breathe in as you shift your weight to the right foot, lift the left heel, turn your body to the right and raise your left hand (palm up).*

7a

**7b**

*Breathe out as you return your body to the front, lower your heel, balance your weight equally on both feet, and lower your hand.*

7b

**85**

## Gazing at the Moon

This movement is an extension of the previous movement. It has a beneficial effect on the shoulder, waist and neck areas, and is particularly recommended for cases of arthritis of the shoulder and weakness of the cervical, lumbar and back muscles.

Also, it benefits the circulation and digestion, and it slims the waist and hips.

### MOVEMENT BREAKDOWN

**Foot- and leg-work**

Stand in the preparatory position. Shift the body-weight to the left foot and turn the body 45 degrees to the left. Return to face the front, with your weight equally on both feet.

Shift the body-weight to the right foot and turn the body 45 degrees to the right. Return to face the front, with your weight equally on both feet.

**Arm-work**

Swing both arms together in a leftward direction until the hands come up above head height (but not over the head) on the left side of the body. The arms should be parallel, with the palms facing out. Look in the direction that the hands point. Lower the arms to the original position.

Then swing both arms together in a rightward direction until the hands come up above head height (but not over the head) on the right side of the body. The arms should be parallel, the palms facing out. Lower the arms to the original position.

When your hands are at their highest point, imagine that you are looking at the moon through the frame of your hands.

### Breathing and coordination

Inhale as you shift the body-weight to the left, turn and swing the arms leftwards.

Exhale as you lower the arms and return to face the front.

Inhale again as you repeat the movement on your right side.

### Energy

The focus is on the *lao gong* point.

*8a*

*Breathe in as you shift your weight to the left, turn your body to the left and raise your hands to the left side. Keep your arms parallel, palms facing out.*

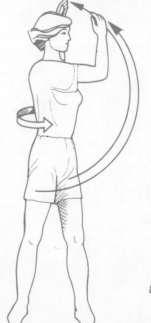

*8a*

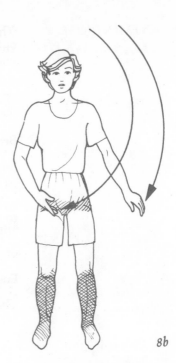

*8b*

*Breathe out as you lower your arms and return to face the front.*

*8b*

## Turning the Waist and Pushing with the Palm

This movement is good for the spleen and stomach functions.

Also, the improved coordination it gives to the muscle groups in the joints and waist can help prevent and cure lumbar muscle strain, and improve the function of the lumbar vertebrae and the lumbo-sacral joint.

It also helps reduce pressure in the cerebral arteries.

### MOVEMENT BREAKDOWN

#### Foot- and leg-work

Begin in the preparatory position. Turn the waist 45 degrees to the right. Return to face the front.

Then turn the waist 45 degress to the left. Return to face the front.

#### Arm-work

With palms facing up, bend the elbows to bring the hands up to hip-level. Push the left palm upwards and outwards till the palm faces forward at chest height.

Simultaneously, turn the right palm over and press down until it is by the side of your hip. Keep the elbows relaxed. Turn the palms up as you draw them back to the initial hip-level position.

Then push the right palm upwards and outwards till it faces forward at chest height. Keep the elbows relaxed.

Simultaneously turn the left palm over and press down. Turn the palms up as you draw them back to the initial hip-level position.

When pushing out, imagine that you are pushing a heavy object away from you.

### Breathing and coordination

Breathe in as you settle the hands by the hips in the preparatory position.

Breathe out as you extend the left palm forward and turn to the right.

Breathe in as you withdraw the palm to the side and return to face the front.

Breathe out you repeat the movement using the right hand.

### Energy

Focus on the *lao gong* point.

As you perform the movement, visualise that you are projecting energy out through your palms.

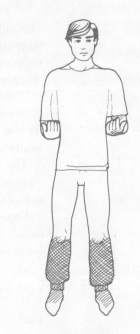

*9a*

**9a**
*Breathe in as you raise your
arms to hip level, palms up and
elbows out.*

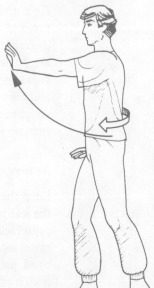

*9b*

**9b**
*Breathe out as you turn to the
right and push your left palm
forward to shoulder height while
you turn the right palm over
and press it down.*

*Breathe in as you bring
your hands back to hip level and
return to face the front.*

*MOVEMENT TEN*
## Cloud Hands in a Horse-riding Stance

The movement from side to side helps strengthen the lumbar muscles, thus reducing the chance of injury or strain in this area.

The deep breathing, turning and lowered stance all contribute to an increased blood-flow to the internal organs, improving their health and function.

The internal massaging effects assist the digestive system, while the arm-work is useful for arthritis of the shoulder.

Focusing mentally on the hands in the clouds helps to raise your emotional balance (*shen*) and focus your willpower (*yi*).

## MOVEMENT BREAKDOWN

### Foot- and leg-work

From the preparatory position, turn the torso 45 degrees to the left, then turn it 90 degrees to the right. All subsequent turns are 90 degrees. Ensure that you turn at the waist and not at the knees. Keep the heels and toes firmly on the ground with the weight equally on both. The spine should turn on its own axis but not bend or sway.

### Arm-work

Keep the palms relaxed throughout. Raise the left hand in front of the face, with the palm facing inwards and the fingers gently extended. At the same time move the right hand, palm-down, slightly out to the side until it reaches hip height, the fingers gently extended.

Reverse the position of the hands until the right hand is raised in front of the face, the palm facing inwards and the fingers extended. At the same time turn the left hand palm-down and lower it to hip height and to the side, the fingers extended.

. As you perform the movement visualise that the hands are moving through the clouds. Indeed, that they are just like the clouds, soft and drifting.

**Breathing and coordination**

Inhale as you bring hands up into position and turn to the left. Exhale as you turn 90 degrees to the right.

Inhale as you exchange the position of

*10a*

*Breathe in as you raise your left hand in front of your face (palm towards you), and move your right hand (palm down) out to the side until it reaches hip height.*

*10b*

*Breathe out as you turn 45 degrees to the left. Your arms should move with the turn of your body so that your position remains aligned.*

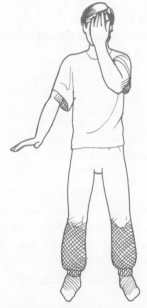

10a

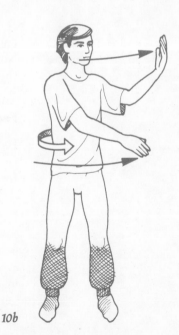

10b

93

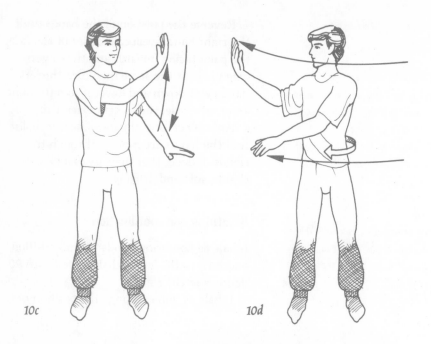

10c

10d

**10c**

*Breathe in as you exchange the position of your hands.*

**10d**

*Breathe out again as you turn to the right.*

hands. Exhale as you turn to the right. Note that the lowered arm should follow the movement of the body.

### Energy

Focus on connecting the *lao gong* and *yin tang* and *tan tien,* so that the energy forms a triangular circuit.

## MOVEMENT ELEVEN
## Scooping the Sea and Looking at the Horizon

This movement involves compression and extension in the vertical, rather than horizontal, axis. This means that the benefits complement those of the previous movement. The overall effects are the same but the two movements enhance each other.

The main benefits of this move are, physiologically, internal massaging and, psychologically, mental balancing. The movement is also particularly useful for stomach problems.

### MOVEMENT BREAKDOWN

#### Foot- and leg-work

Beginning with the preparatory stance, this movement involves two steps.

**Left step:** transfer the weight to the right leg and step forward with the left foot in front of the left shoulder. Move the body forward as you transfer the weight forward, bending the front leg and almost straightening the back leg.

Keep the body upright as you then transfer your weight back to the right leg by bending the right knee and straightening the left knee, then lift the toes of the front foot off the ground.

Then bring the left foot back to the preparatory position.

Throughout the movement, the level (height) of the body should remain even.

**Right step:** transfer the weight to the left leg and step forward with the right foot in front of the right shoulder. Move the body forward as you transfer the weight forward, bending the front leg and almost straightening the back leg.

Keep the body upright as you transfer your weight back to the left leg by bending the left knee and straightening the right knee, then lift the toes of the front foot off the ground.

Remember to keep the level of your body even.

Bring the right foot back to the preparatory position.

## Arm-work

Scoop both hands forward, crossing at the wrists. Lift the crossed wrists up over the head. Separate the hands by pushing them out and then down at your sides, and repeat the scooping. In both the left and right step, place the right wrist over the left.

As you perform the exercise, follow the movement of your hands with your eyes. As you scoop up, visualise scooping up water from the sea. As your hands move upwards, imagine the water falling through your fingers like rain. Then, when your hands are raised, imagine looking into the horizon.

## Breathing and coordination

Breathe in as you move your body forward and bring your arms up.

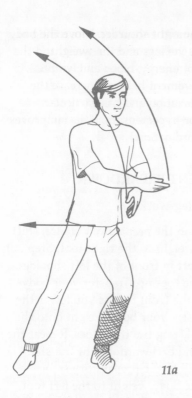

11a

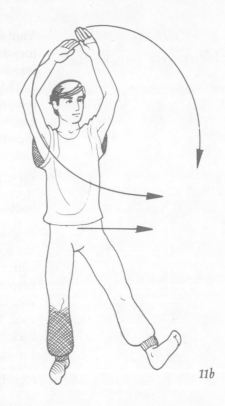

11b

## 11a

*Breathe in as you place your leg in front of you and transfer your weight forward, while simultaneously scooping your hands in front of you and raising them above your head.*

## 11b

*Breathe out as you transfer your weight back onto your right leg (lifting the front toes), and lower your arms back down to your sides.*

Breathe out as you move your body back and lower your arms to scoop.

## Energy

Concentrate on scooping as the body moves forward and on releasing as the body moves back. Focus on raising the energy when scooping and lowering it to the *tan tien* when bringing the arms down.

MOVEMENT TWELVE
## Pushing the Waves

This movement encourages the toning of muscles in the legs and the waist, and the free flow of energy, blood and lymph.

The movement helps to increase the level of relaxation and has particular benefits for hypertension. It also improves muscle coordination.

**MOVEMENT BREAKDOWN**

**Foot- and leg-work**

Beginning in the preparatory stance, shift the body-weight to the right foot. Step out with the left in front of the left shoulder, keeping the toes up. Transfer your body-weight to the front foot as you lower the toes. Transfer your body-weight onto the back foot, lifting the front toes. Repeat the forward and backward weight transfer.

Step back to the preparatory stance.

Shift the body-weight to the left foot. Step out with the right foot in front of the right shoulder, keeping the toes up. Transfer your body-weight to the front foot as you lower the toes. Transfer your body-weight onto the back foot, lifting the front toes. Repeat the forward and backward weight transfer.

Step back to the preparatory stance.

Remember to keep your body level throughout the movement.

**Arm-work**

Raise the hands in front of the body to chest height, elbows down. Then, with palms facing forward at shoulder height, push as far forward as you can without completely straightening the elbows, lifting the shoulders, bending the back or lifting the back heel.

Next, pull the hands back, finishing close to the shoulders but without raising the shoulders.

Relax the chest to lower the hands, then push forward again.

Visualise a wave-like motion as you push forwards and backwards.

## Breathing and coordination

Inhale as you place the left foot forward and lift the hands into position.

**12a**

*Breathe in as you place your left foot in front of you (toes up) and raise your hands to chest height, with your palms facing forward and your elbows down.*

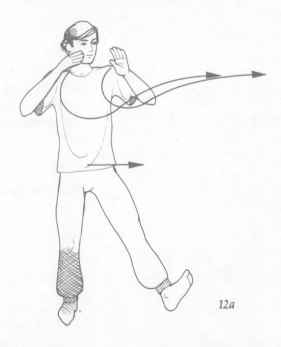

12a

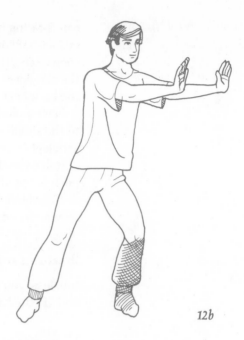

*12b*

*Breathe out as you transfer your weight onto the front foot (lowering the front toes), and push forward with your hands.*

*Breathe in again as you transfer the weight back and draw your hands in toward your chest.*

*12b*

Exhale as you transfer the weight and push forward.

Inhale as you transfer the weight backwards and draw the hands back.

**Energy**

Focus on the *lao gong* point.

## MOVEMENT THIRTEEN
### The Flying Dove Spreads its Wings

The opening and closing of the arms exercises the chest and improves breathing capacity as it helps to dissipate constrictive feelings in the chest. This movement is particularly recommended for breathing difficulties such as bronchitis and emphysema.

It also helps to induce an expansive and relaxed calmness, and is particularly helpful in cases of anxiety or aggressive feelings.

The very deep calming effects of the movement particularly benefit the blood system, and can improve the flow of blood to the heart and brain. It is therefore recommended in cases of cerebral arteriosclerosis and restrictions in blood supply to the coronary artery.

## MOVEMENT BREAKDOWN

### Foot- and leg-work

From the preparatory position, transfer the body-weight to the right foot and step out with the left foot in front of the left shoulder, toes up. Transfer your weight to the front foot and lift the right heel. Then transfer your weight back to the right foot and lift the left toes. Repeat the forward and backward motion, remembering to bend the knee that's carrying the weight.

Step back to the preparatory position.

Transfer the body-weight to the left foot and step out with the right foot in front of the right shoulder, toes up. Transfer your weight to the front foot and lift the left heel. Then transfer your weight to the back foot and lift the right toes. Repeat the forward and backward motion, remembering to bend the knee that's carrying the weight.

Step back to the preparatory position.

Remember to keep the back aligned and the body level during this movement.

### Arm-work

Extend the arms to full width at shoulder height with palms facing forward.

Sweep the arms inwards, still extended, until the palms face each other at shoulder height and shoulder distance apart. Draw the palms in as though holding a large ball against the chest.

Then sweep the arms back out to the side, maintaining their shoulder-height level.

When changing sides, after you have drawn the arms back, lower them to the preparatory position.

Throughout the exercise, visualise a dove spreading and closing its wings.

### Breathing and coordination

Inhale as you take the arms out to shoulder height, put your weight on your right leg and place the left foot in front of you with the toes off the ground.

Exhale as you transfer the weight forward and bring the palms in.

Inhale as you transfer the weight backward and open your arms out to the side.

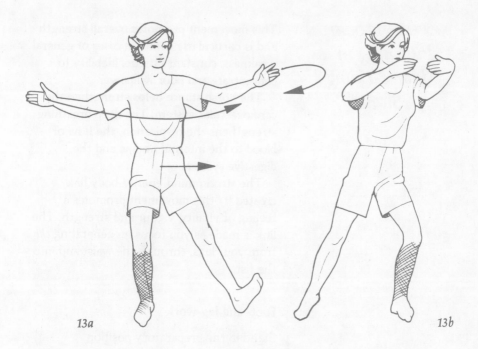

13a

13b

## 13a

*Breathe in as you place your left foot in front of you (toes up) and raise your arms out to your sides (palms facing forward).*

## 13b

*Breathe out as you transfer your weight forward (lowering the front toes) and sweep your arms inward until they are shoulder width apart in front of you.*

*Breathe in again as you transfer your weight and arms back, ready to repeat the movement.*

When changing sides, exhale as you return to the preparatory position.

**Energy**

Concentrate on the *lao gong* point.

MOVEMENT FOURTEEN

# Punching in a Horse-riding Stance

This movement promotes overall strength and is particularly useful in cases of general weakness, constant fatigue, inability to concentrate and poor willpower.

The horse stance helps strengthen the cardiovascular system. The deep breathing strengthens the respiration, the flow of blood to the internal organs and the digestive system.

The strong mind-energy-body link created by this movement promotes a feeling of vitality, vigour and strength. The link is made as you focus on generating *chi* from your legs, through the waist and into the fist.

## Foot- and leg-work

Stand in the preparatory position throughout this exercise. There is no movement of the waist.

## Arm-work

Draw the hands into hollow fists and, bending the elbows, raise the hands to the side of the waist, keeping the knuckles pointing down. Punch forward with the left fist, twisting it so that the knuckles face upwards at chest height. Draw the fist back down to the side of the body, at the same time rotating the wrist to bring the knuckles back to their starting position.

Then repeat the movement using your right hand.

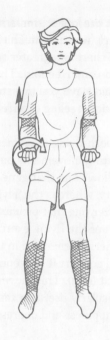

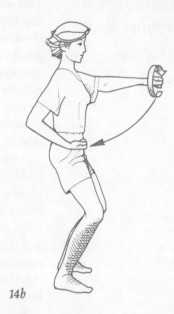

*14a*                                   *14b*

**14a**

*Breathe in as you bend your elbows and raise your fists to hip level.*

**14b**

*Breathe out as you punch forward.*

   *Breathe in again as you withdraw the fist.*

## Breathing and coordination

Inhale as you raise your fists to hip level.
   Exhale as you punch forward.
   Inhale as you withdraw the fist.

## Energy

Focus on the *lao gong* and *tan tien* points.
   Throughout, visualise that you are filling the fist with energy. Concentrate on energy, not force.

*MOVEMENT FIFTEEN*

# The Flying Wild Goose

This movement has lots of similarities to the 'Flying Dove', (Movement Thirteen). Here, however, there is a greater sense of power, expansion and freedom. The movement should leave you in a state of relaxed stimulation, feeling carefree and joyous.

Notice that both flying movements come after *chi*-generating movements but that this exercise follows one that generates a feeling of vitality, whereas the 'Flying Dove' comes after one that promotes relaxation. Each of the flying exercises helps to take energy generated in the body and will (*yi*) and convert it into energy of emotion or spirit (*shen*). This movement is, therefore, particularly useful in cases of long-term unhappiness and depression.

## MOVEMENT BREAKDOWN

### Foot- and leg-work

Stand in the preparatory position. The palms and knees should be relaxed. Raise the body as you lift the heels off the ground and stand on the balls of the feet. Lower the body as you place the heels back on the ground.

### Arm-work

Keeping the arms extended, lift the hands out to the side and then above the head, hands relaxed, palms facing down. Then sweep the palms down to the side again.

In your visualisation, use the image of a large bird flying through the sky.

### Breathing and coordination

Inhale as you take the hands up over the head and raise the body and heels.

Exhale as you bring the hands down to the side and lower the body and heels.

### Energy

The internal focus is on the *lao gong* point. (Keep the eyes looking forward.)

**15a**

*Breathe in as you raise your body and lift your heels as you simultaneously raise your arms to the side until they are well above shoulder height.*

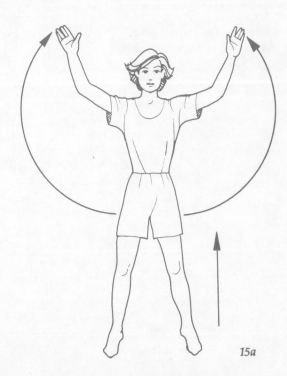

*15a*

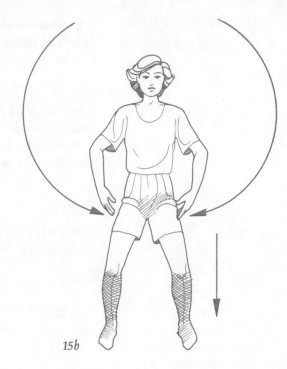

**15b**
*Breathe out as you sink down,*
*lowering your heels, and return*
*your hands to your sides.*

15b

MOVEMENT SIXTEEN
## The Rotating Flywheel

A good circulatory exercise for improving blood, energy and lymph flow. The movement is good for those suffering from low blood pressure, but care must be taken to perform the movement slowly.

It also loosens up the back and shoulders, reducing stiffness and removing tension. The movement tones and stretches the muscles of the back, limbs and waist, helping to prevent the risk of strain and injury. It is also useful (when performed slowly and with care) for aiding recovery from ailments of the cervical and lumbar vertebrae.

**MOVEMENT BREAKDOWN**

### Foot- and leg-work

The movement of your body should naturally follow the movement of your arms: when you raise your arms, your body should rise; when you lower your arms, you should lower your body.

Your body should also follow the arm movement to the left and right, with your head turning in alignment. For example, when you lift your arms on the left side, turn your body to the left; when you lower your arms on the right side, turn your body to the right.

### Arm-work

With palms facing down, raise the arms up to the left, keeping them parallel, until the hands are over the head. Then relax the arms and lower them to the side of the

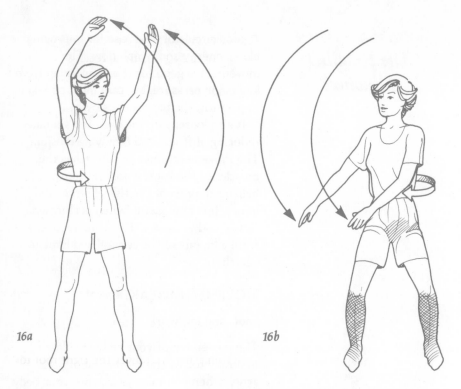

16a

16b

### 16a

*Breathe in as you rise up,*
*taking your arms up above your*
*head and keeping them parallel.*

### 16b

*Breathe out as you sink down*
*and lower your arms on the*
*right side, keeping them*
*parallel.*

body, maintaining their parallel position.

Repeat this large circle in the opposite direction.

As you perform this exercise, visualise the movement of a flywheel.

## Breathing and coordination

Inhale as you rise and take the hands up above the head.

Exhale as you bring the hands down and sink.

## Energy

The internal focus is at the *lao gong* point.

MOVEMENT SEVENTEEN
## Stepping and Bouncing a Ball

This is an invigorating exercise that is useful for raising a general feeling of vitality. It also tends to improve coordination and balance mental functions. The legs are strengthened by taking up the whole body-weight, but they are also relaxed when raised. This exercise gives good opportunity to remove stress in the calf and ankle area.

The movement is recommended for cerebrovascular disease, and conditions of stress and arthritis.

## MOVEMENT BREAKDOWN

### Foot- and leg-work

From the preparatory position, transfer the weight to the left foot and lift the right knee to hip height. Lower the right foot to the ground.

Transfer the weight to the right foot and lift the left knee to hip height. Lower the left foot.

### Arm-work

Raise the left hand to just above shoulder height and then bring the hand down as though bouncing a large ball.

Repeat the movement using your right hand.

### Breathing and coordination

Inhale as you raise the right knee and the left hand.

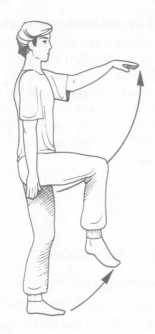

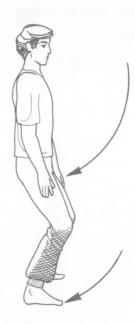

*17a*                              *17b*

**17a**

*Breathe in as you shift the
weight to the left foot, lift the
right knee to hip height and
raise the left arm to shoulder
height in front of you.*

**17b**

*Breathe out as you lower your
arm and leg.*

Exhale as you lower the right knee and
the left hand.

Inhale as you raise the left knee and the
right hand.

Exhale as you lower the left knee and
the right hand.

**Energy**

Focus on the *lao gong* of the lifted hand.

## Balancing the Chi to Close

This technique is a useful one for calming down and may be used independently of the set in cases of stress, tension and emotional unbalance. In addition, it is excellent for reducing hypertension.

### Movement breakdown

### Foot- and leg-work

Commence in the preparatory position. Straighten the knees slightly to rise, then bend the knees slightly to sink.

### Arm-work

Turn the palms outward, then with the elbows moving out to the side, raise the

*18a*

*Breathe in as you turn your palms to face outward, move your elbows out to the side and raise your hands to just above shoulder height in front of you.*

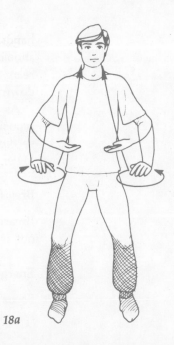

*18a*

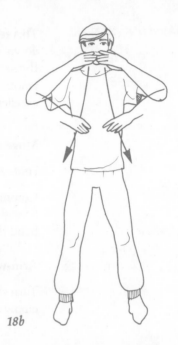

*18b*
*Breathe out as you turn the palms over and lower your hands back to your sides.*

*18b*

hands in front of the body to just above shoulder height. Turn the palms down, relax the elbows and lower both hands down to the side of the body.

As you perform the exercise, visualise scooping up energy from the earth and settling it down through the body as you lower your arms.

### Breathing and coordination

Breathe in as the hands move up. Breathe out as the hands are brought downward.

### Energy

Focus on bringing the energy down the *ren mai* and centring it in the *tan tien*.

*STANDING ZEN*

At the end of the eighteen exercises, perform the 'Standing Zen'. Standing in the preparatory position, relax, keeping the spine straight and place your body weight on your thigh and calf muscles. Place one palm on top of the other on the *tan tien* in a quiet, standing meditation and focus on the *tan tien*.

**Standing Zen**
*Relax in the Preparatory Position, place one palm firmly on top of the other over the* tan tien, *and meditate on the energy in the* tan tien.

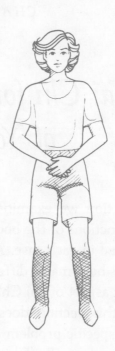

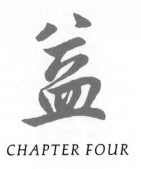

CHAPTER FOUR

# Tai Chi for Specific Parts of Your Body

In this section we examine how Tai Chi can benefit specific parts or functions of the body, detailing the important principles to be applied in each case. As you will see, these principles can be used to help many different health problems, emphasising the holistic aspect of Tai Chi.

While this section does describe specific principles to be applied to specific problem areas, you should keep in mind the holistic aspect of Tai Chi. Each technique explained in this chapter should be integrated into your Tai Chi practice in a balanced way, rather than used exclusively and thus to the detriment of the overall harmony of the body.

Once again, the emphasis is on application of principle rather than on appearance of form. This is especially true for the early stages of your practice, as it is the underlying principles you use, rather than the perfection of the moves, which will dictate the level of benefit you gain.

## HOW TO USE TAI CHI TECHNIQUES TO BENEFIT YOUR HEART, BLOOD PRESSURE AND BLOOD CIRCULATION

In today's stressful life there are few of us who have not experienced, if only secondhand, the fears that arise from heart and blood-pressure problems. The good news is that Tai Chi can be a very effective tool for maintaining our cardiovascular system, normalising blood pressure and improving circulation.

When we think of our blood circulation it is usually in terms of whether our blood pressure is too high or too low. Tai Chi assists in normalising this pressure. A few moments reflection on what the blood system actually does will reveal other benefits which Tai Chi can provide.

Your body is composed of billions of cells. These cells require oxygen and nutrients to survive, and their waste products are toxic and must be removed. This is the job of the blood system. If your blood system is not working properly then the cells become undernourished and poisoned by their own waste products. In such a condition they are easily susceptible to disease.

There is a tendency in the West to see the heart as something separate from the blood circulation. However, we should remember that it is the failure of the blood to circulate that actually kills us, not the stopping of the heart contractions.

It is important to make this distinction because then our

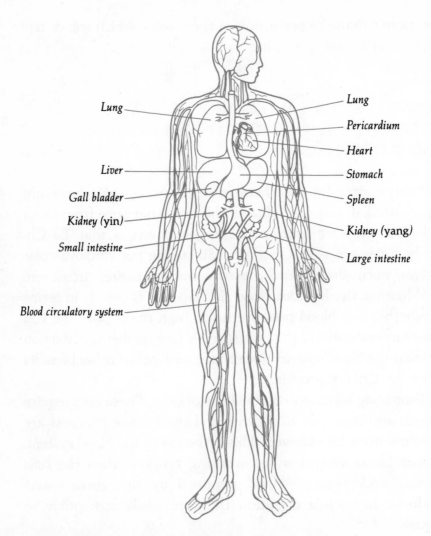

Lung

Lung

Pericardium

Heart

Liver

Stomach

Gall bladder

Spleen

Kidney (yin)

Small intestine

Kidney (yang)

Large intestine

Blood circulatory system

**Figure 5 The Internal Organs and Blood Circulatory System**
*In Chinese medicine and philosophy each organ is either yin or yang, depending on its characteristics and functioning. Yin organs are deep and hidden. They transform, circulate and store chi. Yang organs receive and process food and eliminate waste, and are thus connected to the outside. (The gall bladder, which assists the liver, is the exception. The kidneys possess both yin and yang characteristics and functions.)*

focus is on what makes the blood circulate. There are, in fact, three pumps for the blood system. The heart is the most important, but failure of the other two pumps seriously impairs circulation and brings all the consequent health problems. The three blood circulation pumps are the heart, the musculature, and the lungs. Failure or inefficiency in these other two pumping systems leads to the heart itself having to work far harder than it was designed to, with the consequent risks of failure.

## If you destroy unity
## You destroy yourself.

### The Heart

The heart is like any other muscle: if it works too hard it can be overstrained; if it is not exercised enough it loses the ability to cope with sudden changes in demand. Unlike other muscles, however, we cannot afford even temporary failure of the heart. It is most important that your heart receives the right level of exercise.

The state of your heart is often measured by the number of times it beats per minute. The heart-rate increases for two reasons. First, due to an actual increase in the energy requirements of the body, as occurs during exercise. Second, when the brain receives a stimulus that stresses mental activity sufficiently to activate the 'flight or fight' response.

To deal with a heart rate that is not synchronised with actual body requirements (a stress response), apply the five essential principles of Tai Chi: relaxation, concentration, meditation, harmony and breathing. This section is concerned with the techniques for ensuring that your heart and cardiovascular system have sufficient but not excessive physical exercise.

It may seem curious to talk about exercising the heart when it is always working, but it is the ability of your heart to cope with changes in its workload that is important. Studies carried out to calculate the maximum recommended heart-rate (MHR) find that the most beneficial are exercise levels that raise the heart-rate to between 60 and 80 per cent of the MHR. Such exercises develop the heart's capacity to handle changes in workload, but do not put the heart itself at risk.

Studies carried out in the USA show that performance of Tai Chi in a stance where the knees are considerably bent achieves an increase in heart-rate that falls exactly within the prescribed levels.

Tai Chi is always performed with the knees bent. The more the knees are bent, the higher the cardiovascular loading. In simple terms, the more you bend your knees the more work your leg muscles do, the more oxygen those muscles consume and the faster your heart must beat to maintain the supply of oxygen.

The 60 to 80 per cent loading is quite safe for anyone without severe heart problems and represents the type of loading that one could reasonably expect to occur in day-to-day activities. Inability to cope with such levels could place you at risk, so it is wise to practise an exercise system like Tai Chi to maintain your heart's health.

## Performing Your Tai Chi for the Heart

Start with the knees only slightly bent. You can gradually increase the bend at subsequent practice sessions if there are no adverse symptoms. Remember, Tai Chi is holistic, so do not increase the angle to a point which strains the muscles or distorts the posture. The angle of knee-bend which suits you is completely individual and will change as your health changes. NOTE If you have a serious heart or circulatory condition, or are recuperating from cardiovascular surgery, you should still be able to perform Tai Chi but with your knees only very slightly bent. However, seek your doctor's advice.

---

*Movements which benefit the heart include:* 1. Raising the Arms; 2. Opening the Chest; 5. Rolling the Arms in a Horse-riding Stance; 11. Scooping the Sea and Looking at the Horizon; 17. Stepping and Bouncing a Ball.

---

## The Musculature

As we have seen, the heart is not the only pumping system for circulating blood. Too often, however, it ends up doing nearly all the work, which places it under severe strain.

The veins of the body, particularly in the limbs, are threaded through the muscles. Each time the muscles contract they pump the blood forward, and the veins have their own in-built valves to prevent backflow. If the muscles are not exercised, they lose their tone and become flaccid. In this condition they are useless to pump the venous blood and the heart must use the back-pressure of the arterial blood to shift it. This results in high blood pressure.

If a person is stressed and the muscles are continually held tight, the pumping effect of the muscles is absent and the heart must actually force the blood through them against the muscle pressure. This can also lead to high overall blood pressure.

What you need then is an exercise which tones the muscles, and gently exercises and relaxes them. Tai Chi is perfect for this. (NOTE Building muscle-bulk is in itself irrelevant and can be a health hazard if the muscle-bulk actually restricts blood flow, as can occur after an activity such as weight-lifting is dropped.)

*Performing your Tai Chi for Optimum Effects on Blood Pressure*

There are three main groupings of musculature that need to be considered when working on the 'muscle blood-pump'.

## The legs
Bending the knees during your Tai Chi exercises, works the leg muscles and tones them. It also relaxes them, which is just as important.

You should learn to distinguish *yin* from *yang* in your movements. *Yang* can be seen as the active state of the muscles: when they are contracted and bearing load. *Yin* can be seen as the relaxed state of the muscles: when they are at their natural length and in a resting state.

For instance, when you lift your leg to step, there is no

need for any of the muscles in the lower leg to be contracted; the whole lower leg should feel as though it hangs loosely from the knee. Our mind is often focused on our feet when we walk which causes the raised foot to be held at a slight angle — this tenses the whole lower leg. This tension is avoided when the focus is on lifting and lowering the knees rather than the feet. For this reason, you should 'Walk with your knees'. In other words, learn to use only those muscles which are required for the specific posture and movement you are performing and to relax all other muscles.

The shifting of weight in specific Tai Chi movements is important. The more weight you shift on to one leg, the more work that leg does. This helps to condition the muscles in that leg and to push blood through the venous system. The more weight you shift off the other leg, the more relaxed the muscles of that leg become. This allows the blood to flow more easily into the muscles.

### The limbs generally
The muscles you use to push or kick out are different to the ones that you use to pull in or withdraw. To make sure both sets of muscles are alternately relaxed and loaded during your Tai Chi exercises, focus on the feeling of momentum that rolls outwards and inwards with each move. This will help you to naturally relax and work the muscles.

When you push outwards or pull inwards with the hands you generate a momentum. When cancelling an outward momentum and building an inward momentum, make sure to do this smoothly and slowly to distinguish yin and yang. In your Tai Chi practice, you should never straighten the arms and legs fully. In this way the muscles absorb the momentum rather than the joints, and thus benefit both joints and muscles. By not completely straightening or flexing your joints, you also keep your body relaxed and open for blood to flow freely.

### The back, abdominal and neck muscles

The proper use of these muscles requires more advanced Tai Chi but can be generally explained as follows. When you push forward with your hands you are also pushing backward with your back. So, when you push both forward and upward, so you are actually also pushing backward and downward. This mirrors the pumping and pushing action of the arteries and veins in transporting blood.

In application, simply consider Newton's Third Law of Motion: 'For every action there is an equal and opposite reaction'. In Chinese terms the law might well be rendered 'Every action has its foundation in its equal and opposite reaction'.

---

*Movements which benefit the musculature include:* 3. Painting a Rainbow; 7. Supporting a Ball in Front of the Shoulders; 9. Turning the Waist and Pushing with the Palm; 10. Cloud Hands in a Horse-riding Stance; 12. Pushing the Waves; 16. The Rotating Flywheel.

---

### The Lungs

I have explained how important the muscles are to the proper movement of venous blood. This is all very well for your limbs but what about your internal organs: your liver, spleen, kidneys and so on?

The body has an ingenious system of ensuring that your vital organs are properly supplied with blood — that system is called breathing. Every time you breathe in, your lungs expand and there is less space in the body torso. This means that on the in-breath, the internal organs are gently squeezed of their venous blood. As you breathe out, your lungs contract and the space in the body torso increases. Since nature abhors a vacuum, your internal organs expand to fill that space drawing in the fresh arterial blood.

### Performing Your Tai Chi for the Internal Organs

The proper practice of Tai Chi demands that you breathe correctly. As discussed in Chapters 1 and 2, correct breathing is abdominal breathing (refer to these chapters for further information on breathing). Deep breathing effectively enhances the expansion and contraction of the torso, improving the circulation of blood through the organs and their functioning.

Also, for the lungs specifically, breathing high in the chest does not use the lower lobes of the lungs. This increases the risk of adhesions within the lungs. In our polluted society, it

*Movements which benefit the lungs and internal organs include:* 2. Opening the Chest; 5. Rolling the Arms in a Horse-riding Stance; 6. Rowing a Boat in the Middle of a Lake; 11. Scooping the Sea and Looking at the Horizon.

is important not to allow these pollutants to sit in the lower lobes for extended periods of time, perhaps concentrating to higher levels. Breathing deeply during your Tai Chi practice will help expel these pollutants.


## HOW TO USE TAI CHI TECHNIQUES TO IMPROVE YOUR BODY'S RESISTANCE TO DISEASE

As we have seen, stress and over-exercise reduce the body's capacity to resist disease. (The muscles remain contracted and tense, blood cannot flow as easily and this puts additional strain on our bodies — eventually weakening them.) Tai Chi can not only reduce stress and provide an optimum level of exercise, but it can also directly work on your body's defence systems.

The lymphatic system produces the white cells and antibodies that are such an important part of your defence system. It is also one of the main transport systems for the white cells. Unlike the blood system, movement of lymph is completely dependent on changes in internal pressure caused by body movement and breathing.

The Tai Chi movements which enhance the functioning of the lymphatic system include the following aspects: deep diaphragmatic breathing; musculature movement that alternatively relaxes and loads the muscles; weight transfer and waist movement.

The positioning of the tongue has another interesting impact on the body's defence systems. As both inhalation and exhalation are through the nose, it is possible to keep the tongue resting gently against the back of the upper set of teeth or, if comfortable, even the hard upper palate. Such a position increases salivation and, apart from its digestive effects, saliva contains a quantity of antibodies that help fight airborne bacteria. It is the recommended position for Tai Chi exercises.

---

*Movements which improve your body's resistance to disease include:* 3. Painting a Rainbow; 5. Rolling the Arms in a Horse-riding Stance; 13. The Flying Dove Spreads its Wings; 16. The Rotating Flywheel; 17. Stepping and Bouncing a Ball.

---

## HOW TO USE TAI CHI TECHNIQUES TO IMPROVE YOUR POSTURE

When we think of posture it is usually in terms of whether or not we are holding our back straight. Interestingly, posture has often been associated with attitude and emotion. If we see someone trudging along a street shoulders hunched, eyes downcast, the back tilting forward, it is probably a safe bet that the person is not ecstatically happy. Also, our language is full of images that relate posture and mood: 'Oh he's down today', 'feeling very low', 'really burdened', 'down-hearted', 'low-spirited', 'depressed', 'crushed'. Conversely you might be 'on a high', 'uplifted', 'walking tall' or 'flying high'.

The Chinese view is that posture and mood, like *yin* and *yang*, produce each other, so posture is a part of physical as well as mental health.

# Too hard - you are easily pushed over
# Too soft - you cannot stand.

On a physical level correct posture will help you to avoid or alleviate back pain. Many headaches have their source in incorrect posture, as do a number of digestive problems. Correct posture will help avoid damage to joints. Tai Chi is excellent as a postural correction technique.

Posture is about alignment of all parts of the body, physical and mental. To avoid confusion for the rest of this section I shall substitute the word alignment for posture.

## Alignment of the Head

Hold your head as though it is suspended from a string from the centre or *bai hui* point. Tuck your chin in slightly, relax your jaw and hold your mouth gently closed. Position your tongue behind the teeth, even curled back against the 'wind gate' if this is comfortable. Generally, when you turn, turn your head with your body. Your eyes should follow the movement of your limbs as you focus on the visual imagery of the exercise.

Each alignment has its purpose:

- Lifting your head not only automatically straightens the spine but raises the *shen* (spirit and/or emotional balance). The lifting point of the head, the *bai hui* point, is now the reference point against which the remainder of the body can be aligned.

- Tucking your chin in slightly ensures that you keep your spine aligned. If you push your chin forward you will feel what happens to the spine as it connects with the skull; the neck muscles would also be stressed. Even in our Western culture, a forward thrust chin is associated with pugnacity and aggression — not an appropriate mental posture for Tai Chi.

- Tension is often held in the jaw and needs to be removed. When your tongue is touching the palate, salivation is stimulated. Known in China as 'The Golden Nectar' this saliva aids your digestion and immunological defence systems. It is also now thought to contain hormones, the absence of which lead to premature ageing.

- The eyes are most important. What you see should not solely focus on the thoughts or images of your mind. Your eyes should also be aware of what you are doing, what actions you are performing, so that you can fully express your intent and allow the *chi* to flow and the blood to follow. Nor should you glare through your eyes, staring only at what you are doing or focusing your attention on only one thing. Rather you should express your intent while simultaneously being aware of the activity around you.

This balancing act with the eyes of outward moving expression and inward moving perception is most important to the balance of our emotions and spirit. As human beings we must be aware of both the world and our personal expression within it. On a physiological level this means that we need to retain the use of both our focused and peripheral vision.

## Alignment of the Body Torso

The major alignment you need to achieve is that of the *hui yin* point with the *bai hui*; the balancing of the shoulder and pelvic areas, the tucking in of the buttocks and the 'relaxing of the abdomen'.

The *hui yin* point is at the centre of the perineum (the region between the front and back passages). The alignment of this point to immediately below the *bai hui* point will give your body the correct vertical alignment.

To achieve this alignment, tuck in your buttocks. This is most important as it reduces pressure on the intervertebral disks.

Horizontal alignment occurs with the correct adjustment of shoulders and pelvis. To achieve this, visualise each of these areas as crystal bowls full to the brim with water. Your stance should be such that no water can be spilt in any direction. Make sure the shoulder joints are relaxed.

## Alignment of the Limbs

It is very important that your limbs are aligned correctly. This is most important when you bend your knees. To protect the

All Tai Chi movements work to improve your posture, as they release blocked tension from your body and help you to stand naturally. However, the Preparatory Position and the Standing Zen are particularly beneficial, as your attention is focused on your body rather than on a specific movement, and you can feel any adjustments you need to make in order to correct your posture.

knee joint, the knees should always point in the same direction as the toes when the leg is under load.

As a corollary to the above rule, your toes should never point towards each other when both legs are bent as this will stress the hip joints. For proper circulation, the hip joints should be positioned naturally and the groin area relaxed.

## HOW TO USE TAI CHI TECHNIQUES TO IMPROVE YOUR DIGESTIVE AND ELIMINATIVE SYSTEMS

Before looking at digestion, there is one question often asked about Tai Chi that has a somewhat indirect relation to digestion and that is 'Will I lose weight through Tai Chi?'. The answer is both yes and no.

Tai Chi will burn off some extra kilojoules. However, the Chinese answer to excessive eating is balanced eating. Excessive exercise is not the proper answer to excessive eating. If your over-eating is the result of stress, the relaxation that you obtain from Tai Chi may well result in a reduction of your 'nervous eating' and weight loss may then ensue.

Apart from what you put in it, the functioning of your digestive system is affected by your nervous state, your blood circulation and your physical activity. The benefits Tai Chi brings to your blood circulation and nervous state are dealt with in Chapter 1. These naturally flow on to enhance the digestive processes, but physical activity is also important.

Food is moved along the digestive tract by peristalsis and this action is assisted by breathing and movement. The deep breathing of Tai Chi, along with its waist movement, is of great assistance to the digestive and eliminative systems. Certain movements, such as 'Rolling the Arms in a Horse-riding Stance', may work to directly strengthen your abdominal muscles, increasing the compression and relaxation effect in the abdominal cavity that occurs during breathing.

As noted in other areas, salivation is increased when the mouth is closed and the tongue is resting against the upper palate. Unfortunately because of the nature of the food we eat these days we do not chew enough and chewing is the normal way of stimulating salivation. Saliva contains several enzymes necessary for the proper digestion of food. The increase in salivation is therefore extremely beneficial. (Another way of stimulating salivation is to 'wash the teeth with the tongue'.)

*Movements which improve your digestive and eliminative systems include: 3. Painting a Rainbow; 4. Separating the Clouds; 6. Rowing a Boat in the Middle of a Lake; 8. Gazing at the Moon; 10. Cloud Hands in a Horse-riding Stance.*

## HOW TO USE TAI CHI TECHNIQUES TO BENEFIT YOUR JOINTS

Only when our joints are damaged or injured do we tend to realise how important they are to our quality of life and the activities that we undertake.

A joint is a connection of two or more bones. The connective tissue is generally referred to as cartilage. Friction between the two bones is prevented by fluid contained in a membrane also made of connective tissue.

Problems with the joints generally occur either because the connecting cartilage loses elasticity or because the lubricating membrane cannot function properly due to loss, infection or deterioration of the surrounding bone.

Two things are of critical importance to the health of the joints. These are a proper blood supply and proper exercise.

## Blood Supply to the Joints

Poor blood supply, either as a result of stress or inadequate or improper exercise, is now felt to be a major contributing cause to such conditions as arthritis and rheumatism. Tai Chi reduces the effects of stress on blood supply. It can also, by its continual flowing and relaxed movements, increase the volume of blood passing through the joint.

Blood supply to a joint is restricted whenever the joint is straightened or held at an acute angle. Forming angles with the joints of between 120 degrees and 150 degrees is optimal for blood circulation in the wrists, fingers, elbows and knees (hinge joints). Ball and socket joints (hips and shoulders), around 20 degrees. The ankle is a hinge joint but when standing is generally held at somewhat less than 90 degrees. It is very important when drawing weight back to allow the ankle joint to stretch out to 120 degrees. The 'carry position' of a relaxed foot is also around 120 degrees and it is important for circulation that the foot not be carried in a fixed 90 degree position when walking.

## Exercise for the Joints

Proper exercise includes relaxing your joints to their respective resting angles mentioned in the previous paragraph. A straight leg or an acute angle do not only hinder blood supply; they also increase their vulnerability to damage.

When your joints are straightened they are extremely vulnerable because the connective tissue is stretched and the muscles, being at full contraction and extension, no longer have the ability to cushion any shock and direct it to the body. In this case, the shock must be absorbed completely by the joint. Jumping off a one metre wall, for example, with the knees held in locked position would have disastrous effects. Please do not try this, it is very dangerous! Tai Chi emphasises always holding the limbs with a soft curve, never straight and always leaving something in reserve.

Tai Chi also avoids sudden changes in direction. The momentum of the body is absorbed by the musculature rather than by the joints. Martial arts other than Tai Chi may make exceptions to this rule. A snap kick, for instance, is dangerous because the joint straightens and the only place the momentum of the kick can go is back into the joint. This has been known to rupture the knee joint. Such a situation cannot arise when following Tai Chi principles of movement.

A lack of exercise can result in loss of flexibility and strength of the joint and thus increase the risk of injury. Improper exercise can damage joints, including their membrane and cartilage, and in extreme cases lead to fluid loss. When performed correctly, Tai Chi provides an excellent exercise system to ensure the health of the joints. Its smooth, flowing and relaxed movements work to improve their functioning and condition.

> *Movements which benefit your joints include:* 3. Painting a Rainbow; 5. Rolling the Arms in a Horse-riding Stance; 8. Gazing at the Moon; 11. Scooping the Sea and Looking at the Horizon.

## HOW TO USE TAI CHI TECHNIQUES TO BENEFIT YOUR NERVOUS SYSTEM

The nervous system is designed to integrate the various functions of the body and to allow your body to respond optimally to environmental stimuli.

When you train the mind to focus on a movement, then neural activity in the brain moves from the cerebrum to the cerebral cortex. In stress situations there is often over-excitation of the cerebrum, and therefore Tai Chi can help to ease pressure there.

There are basically two neural systems in the human body: the sympathetic nervous system and the parasympathetic nervous system. The sympathetic nervous system can be regarded as the stimulatory system. It gets the body ready for action. The parasympathetic system relaxes the body and puts it into a resting state. Tai Chi helps to bring these two systems into balance by reducing any stress you may be feeling.

To obtain the benefits of Tai Chi for the nervous system, ensure that you follow the five essential principles of Tai Chi, particularly the aspects of picturing each move and feeling the move as you perform it. Use concentration and awareness as you do the exercises.

> *Movements which benefit your nervous system include:* 1. Raising the Arms; 4. Separating the Clouds; 5. Rolling the Arms in a Horse-riding Stance; 9. Turning the Waist and Pushing with the Palm; 11. Scooping the Sea and Looking at the Horizon; 12. Pushing the Waves; 15. The Flying Wild Goose; 16. The Rotating Flywheel; 18. Balancing the Chi to Close.

## HOW TAI CHI TECHNIQUES CAN BE USED TO BENEFIT YOUR ENDOCRINE AND REPRODUCTIVE SYSTEMS

Both the endocrine system (which is a system of glands, producing hormones and other internal secretions), and the reproductive system are very susceptible to stress or any imbalance in normal neural activity. The correct performance of Tai Chi can harmonise and balance these systems and help to rectify any dysfunction within them.

During Tai Chi practice, the waist and abdomen are well exercised and, as an indirect result, so too are the sex organs. With time and consistent practice, Tai Chi is known to help sexual problems such as premature ejaculation, nocturnal emission, impotence, frigidity and premenstrual tension. As a cultivator of mind and body control, it can also increase your sexual power.

*Movements which improve your endocrine and reproductive systems include:*
3. Painting a Rainbow; 4. Separating the Clouds; 6. Rowing a Boat in the Middle of a Lake; 8. Gazing at the Moon; 10. Cloud Hands in a Horse-riding Stance; 14. Punching in a Horse-riding Stance.

## IMPORTANT POINTS

- Tai Chi is highly effective in maintaining your cardiovascular system, normalising blood pressure and improving circulation.

- There are three pumps involved in circulating blood throughout the body: the heart, the musculature and the lungs. Tai Chi benefits all of these.

- Tai Chi helps your defence system and thus improves your resistance to disease.

- The good posture required in Tai Chi helps your digestive system and joints. It also can alleviate headache and back pain.

- Tai Chi is beneficial in terms of reducing 'nervous eating'. The exercises also burn off excess kilojoules.

- The mobility of the joints is improved by Tai Chi. Exercises combined with moderation in bending and straightening the joints improve blood flow through the joints.

- Tai Chi benefits the nervous system.

- The reproductive system is exercised during Tai Chi practice, and sexual problems can be helped.

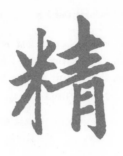

CHAPTER FIVE

# *Incorporating Tai Chi into Your Life*

As I have already stated, Tai Chi benefits you physically, mentally, emotionally and spiritually. I have covered many of these benefits, with emphasis on the physical ones, in the previous chapters. In this chapter, we explore the more general application of Tai Chi in your life.

From the practical concerns of performing your Tai Chi, let's turn to its application in other areas and aspects of your life. This chapter shows you how to incorporate the benefits that flow from both the principles and philosophies of Tai Chi.

Tai Chi is holistic in its approach to health and well-being. It addresses all the needs of the individual, for all influence the individual's state of balance and harmony.

## HOW LONG SHOULD I SPEND DOING TAI CHI EACH DAY?

The simple answer is 'for as long as you enjoy it'. Tai Chi should be one of those activities that you look forward to. However, Tai Chi is not magic. If you perform it in a casual manner for a few minutes a week, don't be surprised if there is no change in the level of your health.

It may only take seconds to relax a muscle but it takes longer to make changes to the body's metabolism and chemistry — especially if these are set at a high stress level. For instance, it may take some time for adrenalin levels in the blood to fall. Modern research tends to indicate that a period of twenty minutes sustained exercise is necessary for significant shifts in biochemical and metabolic activity to take place. I recommend that, at a minimum, you perform your Tai Chi five times per week for continuous twenty-minute periods if you aim at substantial long-term gains in your health.

This does not, however, mean that 'more' is necessarily better in terms of your Tai Chi practice. Your Tai Chi is to be enjoyed. Don't set yourself a practice program that you will not enjoy. If you do, you will find it difficult to gain the relaxation benefits that flow from Tai Chi.

## HOW LONG BEFORE I BEGIN TO FEEL THE BENEFITS OF TAI CHI?

If you approach your Tai Chi with the correct attitude you will begin to feel some of the benefits almost immediately. These are the benefits that flow from relaxing and letting go of the stress that you have accumulated. Other benefits flowing from better muscle tone, deeper breathing, improved posture and enhanced circulation take a little longer to become apparent.

The secret of correct attitude is *play* your Tai Chi! Enjoy yourself. The more *fun* you have with your Tai Chi the more you will benefit your health. Let your Tai Chi work; do not try and make it work. An old Chinese story carries an important message. A keen Tai Chi student approached his master one day and asked him how long under his current training program it would take him to learn his Tai Chi. The master said, 'Oh, about two years.' The student was somewhat depressed and asked what would happen if he doubled his practice time. 'That is difficult to answer' said the master, 'but I would imagine around four years.' The student was aghast and asked what then would happen if he spent every available moment practising his Tai Chi. 'Oh, that's easy' said the master. 'Under those circumstances you will never learn Tai Chi!'

Tai Chi is as much an attitude and an approach to exercise (or life, for that matter) as it is a defined sequence of movements. It promotes harmony, coordination and balance at all levels of your being.

## HOW DO YOU RECONCILE THE PHILOSOPHY OF TAI CHI WITH THE SAYING 'NO PAIN, NO GAIN'?

I don't! Pain has no place in Tai Chi either on a physical or mental level. Pain is your body's warning system, and you disregard that warning at your own risk. Discomfort is another matter. Muscles that have not been used for years may cause discomfort when you begin to exercise them again. A back that is used to sagging forward may not be comfortable when first straightened. On a mental level, if we are trained to use power and force, we may encounter considerable mental discomfort when we try to express slowness and softness.

One of the important aspects of Tai Chi is to learn to distinguish between pain and discomfort. As a good rule, pain tends to be sharp, definite and localised, while discomfort tends to be dull, general and spread over quite a large area. Still, it is best to err on the side of caution. If you feel dizzy or nauseous during your Tai Chi practice, rest immediately. If these symptoms recur, seek medical advice. Discomfort should reduce over time, both on a physical and mental level. Do not be so impatient in your practice that you turn discomfort into pain. Give your body (and mind) time.

Only you can judge whether you are practising too little or too much, too hard or too easy. The act of judging is an exercise in itself that becomes easier as time goes on. It also teaches valuable lessons that can be applied to your whole life. For example, judging how far you can go in a movement also means that you should never over-strain your abilities in other aspects of your life. As the saying goes, you can only do what you can do. However, with practice, you can improve.

NOTE For anyone hooked on the 'no pain, no gain' theory, consider that pain in itself provokes a system-wide response in the body that is equivalent to the stress response. It seems difficult to understand how one can seek health through a response which is directly responsible for ill health!

## TAI CHI AND SPECIAL CIRCUMSTANCES

A natural consequence of Tai Chi's attitude to the 'no pain, no gain' aspect of exercise and its focus on natural movement is that it proves beneficial to the elderly, to sportspeople, to children, to pregnant women, to the mentally handicapped and so on. Just about anybody, no matter what their age or state of health, can do Tai Chi. If, for whatever reason, your health and fitness level concern you, consult your doctor before you begin Tai Chi practice.

### Tai Chi and the Elderly

The proportion of older people in our population is continually increasing. As a result, the health of the elderly should be of growing concern to our society.

If you are elderly, Tai Chi is a slow and gentle form of exercise which can be practised with safety. Even those who consider themselves less fit than their friends of the same age can practise and enjoy the benefits of this art. However, as stated previously, if you are in any doubt as to whether or not a light exercise could be of risk to you, consult your doctor — and this applies especially if you are elderly.

Perhaps the most common and most noticeable effect of old age is poor posture — often the result of a lifetime of bad postural habits. Tai Chi proves highly beneficial in correcting this problem. Along with good posture come all the benefits which are related to it. (These are discussed in Chapter 4 on pages 127 to 131.) In fact, all the benefits of Tai Chi apply just as much to the elderly as to anyone else.

An important aspect to note, however, is revealed in a study titled 'Tai Chi for Postural Control in the Well Elderly'. It showed that elderly people who practise Tai Chi performed significantly better on tests of balance than those who had not practised Tai Chi. Since falling is a common and sometimes fatal problem for the elderly, the balance and postural control gained in Tai Chi could help to reduce the incidence of falling.

## Tai Chi and Sport

Most Australians love the outdoors and sport. The enjoyment we get from outdoor physical activity is a large and important part of the benefits we gain from it. However, often the sports we play have a very aggressive aspect to them. If this aggression is not revealed in the actual playing of the sport itself, it can often be seen in the constant aggressive conditioning we give our bodies. For those who are dedicated, it means hours of struggle — jogging, lifting weights, et cetera.

Worse still, the pressure of winning and getting ahead in a game creates mental pressure and physical tension which is highly detrimental to the body and affects the athlete's flexibilty, movement and performance. Notice how the strongest, biggest, best conditioned or most motivated one is not always the best? It is the one who is also relaxed, nimble in movement, with good ability to concentrate, who is the greatest 'natural' sportsperson. Also required are good breathing ability, balance and coordination. Tai Chi promotes all these things.

To give you an example of how relaxed, natural movement benefits the athlete: in ancient China, the emperor's messengers could run at a steady pace for days on end with little fatigue. What was their secret? The proper alignment of the body combined with a free and natural running action and good breathing technique. The proper posture and movement involves the upper body sitting on top of the pelvis with the abdomen relaxed: the legs do all the action. There should be no effort to pump ahead with the arms. In fact, the arms should be relaxed and hang loosely by the sides of the body until a natural rhythm is established with the momentum of the legs.

With consistent Tai Chi practice you can improve your sports performance, no matter what your chosen sport — tennis, golf, football, basketball, tennis, bowls and so on. Tai Chi will teach you how to hold and move your body correctly, how to relax your mind and body and release tension from the muscles, and it will help you to release untapped energy and vitality — you will play better with less effort and avoid fatigue.

As a complement to training, Tai Chi also works perfectly as a warm up and body toning practice, and it can calm nerves before a game or competition.

## Tai Chi for Children

The growing bodies of children require plenty of movement to help them develop. Playing comes naturally to children, and through play activities they not only exercise their motor coordination, but also learn about interaction with other children and people. The ideal situation is for children to run, climb and play in a healthy, natural, outdoor environment. This not only encourages health but also happiness.

However, in our modern society, especially in cities, space is often limited. The possibility of threat from strangers often forces parents to keep children close by their side. Also, today's busy lifestyles often do not leave much time for parents to take their children to a park or the country to simply enjoy, play and relax.

Even children need to be able to relax from the various stresses they experience in their lives: at school, at home, when Mum and Dad are fighting, when their pet dies . . . In the city, young bodies also have to cope with the effects of pollution. Add on the advent of television and computer games, and it's easy to predict possible results: a sedentary lifestyle, junk food diets, and over-eating are not uncommon.

While children need exercise to develop their bodies, we must realise that the wrong kind of exercise or competitive sport can be very damaging. It is therefore vital to introduce children to suitable physical exercise, and a healthy and balanced lifestyle before bad habits take root.

Tai Chi is suitable for people of all ages and physical ability. For children, the movements not only exercise their torso and limbs, but also improve their motor coordination. Tai Chi promotes good posture, strength and suppleness. Also, children's imaginations are fertile ground for the mental imagery of the movements — and they find them fun.

A survey conducted by the Australian Academy of Tai Chi to establish the benefits of Tai Chi for school children gave very positive results. Teachers of seven to thirteen year olds reported calmness, improved attentiveness and overall better behaviour in class. Tai Chi has also helps children to overcome writing difficulties. Of course, children can also enjoy the other many benefits of Tai Chi: its positive effects on insomnia, asthma and headache just to name a few.

## Tai Chi and Pregnancy

Exercising during pregnancy can be of great benefit. The problem for expectant mothers is finding a form of exercise which is safe for both mother and baby. Tai Chi is an ideal way of keeping fit, supple and relaxed when pregnant. There are no harsh, strenuous or jerking movements, no heavy breathing (panting) and no over-exertion when bending or twisting. If you are pregnant, Tai Chi can gently and safely help you to prepare for the beautiful, even though often painful, experience of childbirth.

Good posture is always important and even more so during pregnancy. Many pregnant women suffer lower back pain caused by extra abdominal weight throwing greater strain on the back. Tai Chi promotes good posture and eases the problems associated with poor carriage.

Tai Chi also helps to strengthen the thighs. This is of particular benefit, as during pregnancy lifting heavy objects is often difficult. It is advisable that you keep your back straight. When you do need to bend, bend from your knees, making sure your thighs do all the work.

Swollen ankles during pregnancy can be caused or exacerbated by poor circulation. Tai Chi, for reasons discussed in previous chapters, encourages the proper circulation of blood throughout the body and can thus help ease this problem.

The art of relaxation is one of the major benefits which even beginners in Tai Chi experience almost immediately. Being relaxed will obviously help you during pregnancy. You will especially find proper breathing (abdominal breathing) of help during your labour. Breathing deeply also aids the nourishment of mother and baby.

The arm movements of Tai Chi help build strength in the arms and upper body, conditioning and preparing these areas for when you need to carry your child. It also tones all the muscles of your body, including the abdominal muscles. Continued Tai Chi practice can assist you in regaining shape slowly and naturally after the birth.

The meditation involved in Tai Chi is also very beneficial in warding off postnatal depression.

Many gynaecologists and obstetricians are in favour of Tai Chi because of its gentle nature. However, you should check with your doctor before practising Tai Chi during pregnancy.

## Tai Chi and the Mentally Handicapped

The slow and gentle movements of Tai Chi are easily learnt by people who are mentally handicapped. The exercises prove highly effective in helping them develop their physical and mental abilities.

Physically, Tai Chi increases awareness of their bodies and coordination. Mentally, it improves their attention spans and concentration. Emotionally it helps them to centre themselves, and the joy of accomplishing the movements brings confidence.

There are some organisations for mentally handicapped people which run Tai Chi classes. The Challenge Foundation and the Wind Gap Foundation are two. Check if similar organisations near you run classes.

## BALANCING YOUR LIFESTYLE WITH TAI CHI

When we look around we can see that balance of body and mind does not always occur. Particularly in our fast-paced, success-oriented world, people often focus on one thing in their life to be the best, rather than working on balancing the whole person. For some intellectuals, the mind is used for rational thoughts and creativity; the body often merely a vehicle to serve the mind. For some others, concern about the body is an obsession: high heels, fad diets, gym workouts and so on, ignore the harmony that needs to be achieved between the body and mind for overall health to result.

Tai Chi exercises the body, mind and spirit (*chi*) in unison and brings out the natural abilities of the whole person.

### Balance is also a State of Mind

Balance is the key to all Tai Chi postures and movements. In life, when things are balanced, there is stability; when not, things become rocky. To give you an analogy: sailing in a boat on the sea is a pleasant experience. However, when the wind picks up, the waves rise and we are buffeted about, it is another experience altogether. Our adrenalin rises (the stress response) and our bodies prepare for immediate action. Some may even enjoy the thrill of a dangerous adventure — yet with the hope or belief that they will eventually escape it.

Thoughts and emotions can sometimes seem like a rocky or even a raging sea. Yet, unlike the sea, you can gain control of your thoughts and emotions. You can calm them so that you can direct your course, clearly and steadily. You can enjoy your journey, reach your destination safely and then rest rather than repair any extensive damage. To achieve this, you need balance. You need to coordinate the various aspects of yourself (mind, body, spirit) and your life (home, work, social, et cetera).

We live in a time of uncertainties. In the current situation of the world, everything seems to be in a state of flux . . . economic upheaval, changing technologies, war, famine, AIDS, changing values . . . We fish around and grasp at different models and theories for some sense of equilibrium. Yet there is only ever one certainty: everything changes.

Life is constantly changing. Changing is Nature's key for survival. If a creature cannot adapt to a new environment, it dies. Life is change. Given this, we must move and change with it if we are to live.

Amongst all this change we can, however, find stability. Tai Chi seeks this 'stillness in movement'. Every Tai Chi movement expresses balance and stability. When things are balanced, they all work together for the benefit of the whole — in this case, you. The practice of Tai Chi is the beginning. The balance you will gain as your body, mind and spirit work in harmony will flow over into other aspects of your life. Just why and how is discussed in the following sections of this chapter.

## Harmony

Harmony is the quest of the Tai Chi practitioner. With harmony there is no sense of division, no struggle or conflict. Within yourself there is a very peaceful feeling, engendering satisfaction and safety. This further enhances your state of relaxation, calmness and softness.

An extension of this philosophy is the harmony you can achieve with other people and your environment. With a calm and open mind, you can respond appropriately to the challenges and trials that come your way. You can also fully appreciate the myriad of people and things around you.

## THE SPIRITUAL BENEFITS OF TAI CHI

The Taoist view of the universe is organic, where all things are connected and intertwined. The cosmos is seen as an inseparable reality — forever in motion and alive, both physical and spiritual. All life is connected through the spirit, the same spirit that breathes life into you also gives life to everything around you. In Taoist understanding, you are not a separate part of the universe but intimately connected with it.

Based on this understanding, your Tai Chi practice gives you greater awareness which can open your mind not only to the life within you but also the life around you.

The balance and harmony that the proper practice of Tai Chi brings can be reflected in every aspect of your life.

### Moderation

Tai Chi teaches moderation. No Tai Chi movement is ever strained. No limb is ever extended completely straight, nor is it ever completely bent. All movements are soft and rounded, leaving something in reserve. Just as in the example where if you jump from a one-metre-high fence with your knees straight you physically injure yourself, so too do you risk injury to your mental, emotional or spiritual state if you strain them to your maximum effort.

You need to remain open and flexible if you are to accept new people, ideas, et cetera. This cannot happen if all your energy and attention is already taken up. If your effort is strained, your perception becomes blocked by tension and you can miss many valuable aspects of the life going on around you. You need to remain open and receptive in order to see the whole picture. Just as the trees must not stand rigid but rather bend with the wind to survive, so too must we.

## Concentrate on the Present

In Tai Chi, through the practice of focusing your attention, you learn to concentrate on the present, not dwell on the past or dream of the future. Attention on the here and now promotes acceptance.

Only by giving your complete attention to each Tai Chi movement will those movements be strong, clear and beautiful to do and to watch. Inattention makes the movements careless, sloppy and boring. So too must you pay attention to the here and now in your life.

## Be Aware of What is Going on Around You

In your Tai Chi movements you are taught to focus on your visualisation, but never to the extent that you are not totally unaware of what is around you. In life, you also need to be aware of other life around you. When driving a car, the ability to drive the vehicle is automatic. However, while you concentrate on the road in front of you, you still need to be aware of any traffic and pedestrian activity around you. If your mind is engrossed in other thoughts, the possibility of an accident occurring increases.

If you are experiencing difficult times, Tai Chi can help you to cope with the stress as you work your way through problems. It will help to ease the turmoil inside you so that you can keep going. The knowledge that you can cope, that you can calm rough waters, will help you to accept reality and deal with it. Tai Chi teaches you to concentrate on one thing at a time and to trust that you will be able to cope with any obstacles that come your way. This not only breeds self-confidence but also peace of mind.

## Let Go

In your Tai Chi practice you will at first need to use your mind to control your physical and mental state. Eventually, you will learn to simply 'let go'. According to Taoist doctrine, thought and desire prevent relaxation. It is only when we stop trying and act spontaneously that we are truly relaxed.

Many things prevent us from acting spontaneously. Two of them are disturbing thoughts of the past or future and our entire past conditioning. There are many things that influence how and what you think. Your upbringing, your social and political background, your economic situation and your cultural heritage all condition your mind to think in certain ways. Rather than helping you to understand things, these conditions can sometimes limit your perception. Prejudice and a closed mind result. This prohibits you from free and natural thought.

As long as your mind is burdened with the beliefs of the past, it cannot be sensitive to the present, and as a result you bring your past experiences and prejudices to a totally new situation — whether appropriate or not. Tai Chi helps you to relax, concentrate on the present and let go. In doing so, it encourages an open mind.

The philosophy behind Tai Chi and the practice of the art itself will help you gain self-acceptance. If and when you feel fear, emotional pain, loneliness, you will recognise their source as attachment to people, things, ideals. Tai Chi will help you to learn to let go as it releases your mind from nagging bonds and centres it on the balanced, soft and gentle movements of your body. If anything, it will teach you that you don't have to feel something as badly or as greatly all the time. The dynamic meditation of Tai Chi can ease your mind, if only for a little while each day. Gradually, this time will increase.

## Don't be Afraid to Be You

In *The Tao of Pooh*, Benjamin Hoff tells the story of Winnie-the-Pooh in the light of Taoism. Pooh is shown as the example of one who follows the Tao: 'Pooh just is'. As a result, he is the most useful person of the group of friends. His mind isn't caught up in the past or future, in dwelling on thoughts, but is calmly focused on what is happening around him.

*Do you want to be really happy? You can begin by being appreciative of who you are and what you've got. Do you want to be really miserable? You can begin by being discontented. As Lao-tse wrote, 'A tree as big around as you can reach starts with a small seed; a thousand-mile journey starts with one step.' Wisdom, Happiness, and Courage are not waiting somewhere out beyond sight at the end of a straight line; they're part of a continuous cycle that begins right here. They're not only the ending, but the beginning as well. The more it snows, the more it goes, the more it goes on snowing.*

Another term for the stress response could be the 'fear response'. We become mentally stressed because we are afraid. Our response to this is active — fight or flight. As discussed in previous chapters, this response is appropriate in certain situations but not in all. When our stress response has nowhere to go, it remains locked within us. The instinctive choice of 'fight or flight' is pulling at our minds and bodies to act but, as it is inappropriate and thus left unresolved, we become confused.

Trying to be what you want to be rather than being who you are, trying to change an unchangeable situation rather than changing your response to it causes confusion and stress. 'Why aren't things working as they should? I'm doing all I can.' The answer is to STOP doing. Relax. Let your mind calm down and then calmly think about things.

Though we have spoken of acceptance and calmness, Tai Chi does not teach passivity. It does, however, encourage movement and change. Tai Chi teaches that change can be coped with and is, in fact, a natural and essential part of life. Tai Chi makes you aware and responsive to what is happening around you. If you are in harmony with this, then you can know and do what is appropriate. All you need to do is take the first step. With each step, the next will become easier and easier.

## Be Calm and Empty

In Chapter 2, I spoke about the state of *Wu Chi*: the ancient Chinese belief that in the beginning, the world was void and boundless. From this arose activity (*yang*), and the state that includes both activity and inactivity (*yin*) was called Tai Chi. Tai Chi teaches you to regain inactivity in your life. When all seems stressful and chaotic around you, Tai Chi helps you to return to the beginning — boundless *Wu Chi* makes all things possible. It symbolises a free and peaceful mind, one that is open to the world around it and can therefore clearly see what is happening and respond appropriately.

In the doctrine of Taosim, the 'Uncarved Block' is the self before it is altered by conditioning, experience and learning. It is the self 'unmade', ready to be made new. Tai Chi helps you to return to the state of the 'Uncarved Block' as it frees you from all prejudice, conditioning, et cetera and allows you to just be.

Gaining the constancy of *Wu Chi* as an 'Uncarved Block' brings balance and stability to your life. Only by emptying yourself of everything will you gain wholeness (the harmony of body, mind and soul), and only when you are empty can you receive. When this is the foundation from which your life springs, then you will be strong.

*Empty yourself of everything.*
*Let the mind rest at peace.*

*The ten thousand things rise and fall while the Self watches their return.*
*They grow and flourish and then return to the source.*
*Returning to the source is stillness, which is the way of nature.*
*The way of nature is unchanging.*
*Knowing constancy is insight.*
*Not knowing constancy leads to disaster.*
*Knowing constancy, the mind is open.*
*With an open mind, you will be openhearted.*
*Being openhearted, you will act royally.*
*Being royal, you will attain the divine.*
*Being divine, you will be at one with the Tao.*
*Being at one with the Tao is eternal.*
*And though the body dies, the Tao will never pass away.*

Lao Tsu

When your mind, body and spirit are in harmony you will find life much easier. You will be integrated and whole, and life will be easier and much more enjoyable. A whole person has an open mind and can place each of life's challenges in perspective and know how to respond. Tai Chi can help you get there.

*IMPORTANT POINTS*

- The philosophies and principles of Tai Chi can be applied to all aspects of your life.

- Your Tai Chi practice should last as long as you enjoy it. At a minimum, twenty minutes, five times a week.

- The saying 'no pain, no gain' has no place in Tai Chi.

- Tai Chi can be safely practised by the elderly. It can also improve your performance in sport and children's health, fitness and ability at school. It can help ease pregnancy and labour and bring joy to the mentally handicapped.

- Tai Chi exercises the mind, body and spirit, and brings out the natural abilities of the whole person.

- Tai Chi can help you to balance your thoughts and emotions and be calm.

- Life is constantly changing, but Tai Chi can help you find stability.

- The calmness, relaxation and stability you acquire in Tai Chi will help you to open your mind to the life within and around you.

- Apply the concept of moderation in all you do.

- Give your attention to the present.

- Tai Chi will help you to learn to let go.

- Be calm, be yourself. Don't strain to be someone else.

- Tai Chi helps you return to the state of the 'Uncarved Block'. This state of freedom and emptiness makes all things possible.

# Glossary

**Buddhism:** teaches that desire brings sorrow and that the annihilation of desire brings peace and ultimately Nirvana.

**Chi (Qi):** literally means 'energy'; usually refers to 'life force' or 'innate energy'.

**Confucianism:** philosophy of humanism which concentrates on world of living (rather than spiritual needs or next world); advocates an ethical system based on justice, moderation and adherence to traditional values.

*I Ching (Book of Changes):* name and rationale of book refer to the concept of constant change which is the result of the interaction of *yin* and *yang*.

**Meditation:** involves experiencing moments of inner stillness; vital to mental and physical well being.

**Meridians:** an invisible network of pathways and channels along which the *chi* flows; links *chi*, blood and fluids. Two major meridian paths are the *ren mai* and *du mai*. Major meridian points include: *yong quan, lao gong, bai hui, hui yin, yin tang, shanz hong, qi hai, ming men* (see Figure 4, page 39).

**Naturalism:** doctrine of Taoism which recognises the soft, yielding and changing ways of nature, and teaches that happiness and longevity are achieved by following the laws of nature.

**Qigong (Chi Kung):** literally *qi* means 'energy' and *gong* means 'skill'; refers to the practice of Chinese energy meditation where *chi* is cultivated.

**Shibashi:** a set of eighteen Tai Chi exercise techniques for cultivating health and energy.

**Stress:** feelings of tension, anxiety, frustration, et cetera caused by the stress-response forcing the body's functioning into an excited, imbalanced state.

**Stressor:** that which activates the stress response, for example, physical danger, arguments, et cetera.

Stress-response: termed 'flight or fight' response, and triggered when stressors activate body systems to function at an intensive level; can be beneficial for short-term defence against physical danger.

Tai Chi: full name is Tai Chi Chuan which means 'Supreme Ultimate Fist'; rather than referring to the combat fighting methods from which it developed, Tai Chi usually refers to health and relaxation exercises (and the unity of *yin* and *yang*).

Tan Tien: literally 'field of breath'; an area about three finger widths below the navel which represents the centre of gravity when the body is relaxed. *Chi* is stored in the *tan tien*.

Taoism: doctrine taught by Lao Tsu which advocates Naturalism and emphasises effortless action to achieve peace, harmony and longevity.

Uncarved Block: in Taoist doctrine, denotes humans pristine state of existence before they were tainted by conditioning, experience and learning. To attain fulfillment, one must become as an uncarved block.

Visualisation: in Tai Chi it refers to the mental imagery of the movement you are performing; increases concentration and links the mind, body and spirit (*chi*).

Wu Chi: literally, 'nothingness'; the boundless void which existed at the beginning of time from which *yin* and *yang* arose.

Yin/Yang: literally *yin* means 'shady side' and *yang* means 'sunny side'; concept that everything is divided into opposite and mutually dependent parts.

# Bibliography

Bailey, Diana M. and Tse, Shuk-Kuen, 'Tai Chi and Postural Control in the Well Elderly', *The American Journal of Occupational Therapy*, Vol. 46, No. 4, April 1992, pp. 295-299.

English, Jane and Feng, Gia-Fu, translators, *Lao Tsu: Tao Te Ching*, Vintage Books, New York, 1972.

Hoff, Benjamin, *The Tao of Pooh*, Methuen Childrens Books, London, © Benjamin Hoff 1982.

Selye, Dr Hans, *Stress Without Distress*, Harper & Row Publishers, Inc., New York, 1974.

# Index

# ACKNOWLEDGMENTS

Researching and writing this book was not a simple task. Many people contributed time, information and suggestions that not only made this book possible, but also greatly enriched it.

I would like to thank the following people for their generous help and encouragement: Rod and Kim Ferguson, David Walker, Jill Wayment, Sandra Selig, Ruth Reeks, June Williams, Byllye Green and Judy Moore.

With special thanks to: J. J. Attenborough and Kirsty Melville for their faith and foresight; Narelle Segecic for her outstanding editing, dedication and support; and Dr Garry Egger for contributing the Foreword.